Frankincense & Myrrh

Also by Wanda Sellar
THE DIRECTORY OF ESSENTIAL OILS

WANDA SELLAR & MARTIN WATT

Frankincense & Myrrh

Through the Ages
and a complete guide to their
use in herbalism and aromatherapy today

Indexes Compiled
by Lyn Greenwood

SAFFRON WALDEN
THE C.W. DANIEL COMPANY LIMITED

First published in Great Britain in 1996
by The C.W. Daniel Company Limited
20 Vauxhall Bridge Road
London
SW1V 2SA

ISBN 9780091955731

The Random House Group Limited supports The Forest Stewardship
Council® (FSC®), the leading international forest-certification organisation.
Our books carrying the FSC label are printed on FSC®-certified paper.
FSC is the only forest-certification scheme supported by the
leading environmental organisations, including Greenpeace.
Our paper procurement policy can be found at
www.randomhouse.co.uk/environment.

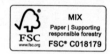

Produced in association with
Book Production Consultants plc,
25-27 High Street, Chesterton, Cambridge, CB4 1ND, England

Printed and bound in Great Britain by
Clays Ltd, St Ives plc

DEDICATED TO

Bernie and Sue

Contents

THE INCENSE TRAIL

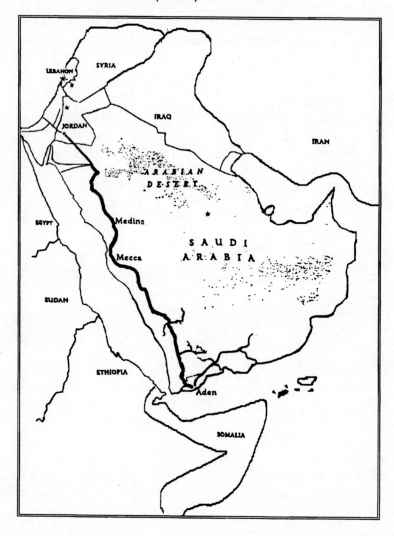

FOREWORD

The idea for this book was conceived soon after a trip to Tunisia. Our goal was to visit essential oil production areas, but we also had time to wander amongst the ruins of Carthage – once the centre of the Phoenician Empire. Amongst the fallen rock and ballista balls, we saw the crimson vetch growing amongst the cypress and eucalyptus. Here and there were yellow-green umbels of caraway or fennel and fig trees growing out of stone walls. Yet the most arresting sight amongst the ruins was the startling yellow of the mimosa trees, the tiny yellow pompons arranged in elongated clusters spreading like sunshine through the pinnate leaves.

Here was splendid evidence of an ancient herb garden. Over the centuries, these herbs and plants of various shapes and colours seeded themselves amongst the ruins and had brought a spark of the past into the present. It was a whimsical notion of course, but as we surveyed the colourful profusion of plants, we imagined them standing as silent witnesses to the events of history.

It would be interesting, we thought, to chronicle the history of some celebrated plant and see how it had influenced civilisation 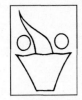 throughout the ages. Somehow the name of frankincense suggested itself, and who can refer to this well-known aromatic without also referring to myrrh? These plants have many associations. The ancient pyramid vaults, the great religions and the three gifts bestowed on Jesus, conjure up so many fascinating images. Of course, frankincense and myrrh were also used extensively in healing.

A Hieroglyph for Incense

We were amazed how much information there was on these plants – but you had to know where to look for it. First-class botanical and historical information was to hand, though much of it was quite technical. We have tried to draw together the strands of information, to provide a comprehensive picture of how these resins have been utilised by mankind over thousands of years. This process has been tremendously enhanced by recent scientific research, which is indicating that aromatic plants do indeed have potent effects on our emotional and physical health. Of course our predecessors knew that thousands of years ago.

However, since the book may be of general interest to the public as well as practitioners of the healing arts, a glossary of terms is given at the back. We have also tried to reference our material in as much detail as possible.

To commemorate our journey through the clouds of incense, we have also made our own 'Meditation Blend' and named it 'Lebonah'.

History

'Until the day break, and the shadows flee away
I will get me to the mountain of myrrh,
And to the hill of frankincense.'
Song of Solomon 4:6

Which other aromatics fire the imagination more than the legendary frankincense and myrrh? They were the most prized aromatic gums of the ancient world and a significant source of wealth in southern Arabia. Their universal appeal has remained constant throughout the ages; surely a testimony to their intrinsic worth.

Was it ancient man who, back in the distant past, first discovered the haunting fragrance of frankincense and the smoky notes of myrrh? When he threw the twigs on the camp fires, did their aromas lull him to sleep? It is possible too that their preservative properties may first have been observed when insects were found in the resin masses, perfectly preserved. Perhaps when hands were grazed and cut gathering wood, their wound-healing properties were first noticed.

Aromatic gums, like frankincense and myrrh, developed into a precious commodity in the ancient world and their use, particularly in the form of incense, goes back to a period of extreme antiquity. 'Incense' referred to the aromatic smoke rising from any odiferous material burned over hot coals, but throughout the centuries the word became synonymous with frankincense – meaning 'true incense'.[1] It was prized above all other resins except myrrh – which was three times as valuable – but frankincense generated five times the demand of myrrh.

Why were frankincense and myrrh so popular? Was it due to their superior aroma or perhaps because of their fixative value – giving a lasting quality to a perfume blend? Or could it be that the pervading strong smells of those times needed fragrant herbs and spices to mask unpleasant odours and keep vermin and insects at bay? Both resin gums had many uses: in perfumery, as varnishes and in medicine.

The magical frankincense was actually derived from the resin of a rather unspectacular scrubby tree found growing in the arid regions of Arabia and East Africa. Despite its lowly origins the world clamoured for its share of this beautiful resin which was used in perfumery, healing and worship. The name frankincense is derived from the Old French:

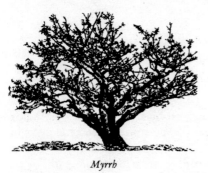

Myrrh

franc meaning free, pure or abundant, and the Latin *incensum*, to kindle. It is also known as *olibanum* from the Arabic *luban* (referring to the milky juice exuding from the tree) although both frankincense and myrrh, as well as other balsam trees, were often referred to as luban. The Hebrews called it *lebonah*.

The myrrh tree has the same unprepossessing appearance as frankincense, nevertheless, it seems to appeal to goats who feast in the prickly shrublands, and carry off myrrh globules on their beards. These are combed off, as we are led to believe, and sent to the market. (Apparently both myrrh and frankincense are said to make excellent fodder for both goats and camels.) Myrrh tends to grow all over southern Arabia but the principle growing areas appear to have been between modern Bayhan and Shabway. The true myrrh was often sold in markets under the name of *karam* to distinguish it from the opaque bdellium known as *meena harma*. Bdellium, probably *Commiphora africana*, was an inferior myrrh and often mixed with the true myrrh or sometimes substituted for it. Dioscorides opined the variety called *Troglodytica* to be the best. Myrrh is first mentioned in Exodus 30:23, and often referred to as *mor* or *myr*, a derivative from the Arabic *murr* meaning bitter.

It is supposed that frankincense and myrrh were used for the first time in ancient south Arabia. Archaeological evidence shows scripts on sherds found in Eilath dated to the fifth or sixth centuries BC. This is the earliest archaeological evidence of the incense trade.[2] A relief from the collection of South Arabian antiquities gathered by C. Rathjens Sabaeica, II, (Hamburg 1955, p.109 and 247, phot. 399) represents an offering-scene in front of an incense altar. Also, an hellenistic bronze

statuette of a woman offering incense has been found in the Wadi
Shalala and is now preserved in the National Museum in Sana under the
signature YM 289. There is archaeological evidence for the use of
incense in Palestine and Syria in the second millennium BC. At Megiddo
elaborate pottery incense bowls on tall stands were found in a stratum
dated to the 11th century BC, while a horned limestone incense altar is
attributed to a stratum of 1050–1000 BC.[3] It is not entirely clear
however, whether the incense used was frankincense or myrrh or
whether it came from south Arabia.

Indeed, excavations have unearthed incense burners in great
numbers in southern Arabia.[4] The south Arabian texts frequently
mention incense offerings in domestic sanctuaries, though many incense
burners have been found at the excavations of burial-places. The
incense offerings were presented on small cube-shaped altars which
have a cavity on top and four short legs or a
quadrilateral base.

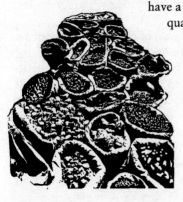

Theophrastus was probably the
first to provide an eye-witness
account of incense trees growing
in south Arabia. This was by using
the reports of reconnaissance
vessels sent out by Alexander the
Great. In *Enquiry into Plants*
Theophrastus mentions that the
harvested myrrh and frankincense,
which was destined to be sold, was
first brought to the temples of the
gods. The resins, bundled and labelled, awaited the merchants who
came to buy whichever bundle pleased them. A third – or according to
Pliny *(Naturalis historia XII, 63)* a tenth part of the harvest was
appropriated by the priests who seem to have exercised a monopoly in
the trade. Indeed this is revealed in an epigraphic text, CIH 400, which
is engraved on the pillar of a temple in Marib, clearly expressing the
prohibition of taking away from the sanctuary or intercepting any
incense of the sun-god.[5] Obviously, frankincense was sacred
to the gods and according to Theophrastus, particularly
sacred to the sun-god.

Chief importers of the resins were Egypt, Persia,
Babylon, Assyria, Greece and Rome. Herodotus (c.300 BC),
the Greek historian and traveller, describes the yearly
BAAL
tribute of a thousand talents (ancient unit of weight and

money) of frankincense to the Babylonian king Nebuchadnezzar. This amounted to 98,422 lbs. The incense was burned at the altar in the great temple erected to the honour of Baal.

A similar amount was paid in tribute by the Arabs to the Persian king Darius (c.496 BC), no doubt in honour of his many conquests.[6]

Yet what was the significance of using resins like frankincense and myrrh in worship to god and king alike? Apparently it was thought that the smoke rising heavenwards from the sweet burning incense forged a symbolic link between the people and their gods. The burning of incense on more secular occasions is described by Herodotus. In the procession organised by Antiochus Epiphanes, king of Suria (Syria), at the Daphen sports, great golden dishes filled to the brim with myrrh and frankincense were carried by a cortege of young boys whilst the guests were sprinkled with scented water. Another procession followed with a golden altar, accompanied on either side by an incense burner made of ivy wood and gold.[7]

The use of frankincense and myrrh was, of course, not restricted to worship or aesthetic adornment. Since aromatics were derived from natural materials, their medicinal value was immense. Most of the ancient texts on medicines, perfumes and incense, from about 4000 BC onwards, included frankincense and myrrh. These can be found in the early Syriac Herbals, Egyptian Texts (both carved hieroglyphs and papyrus), Biblical books and in Greek and Roman works. The Chinese, as far back as the 10th century, also imported frankincense from Arabia for medicinal use. The Chinese burned incense before they consulted their oracle book the *I Ching*. Though trading routes existed with the Arabian world, it is not known whether they used frankincense from India or from Arabia.

In fifth and sixth century the healers in India burnt incense sticks to subdue the demons that were causing problems for people suffering from arrow wounds. Once these evil spirits were driven away then the life of the patient was spared.

The Incense Route

Southern Arabia's wealth in ancient times rested very much on skilled irrigation schemes and agriculture. Yet it is also true to say that part of that country's wealth – and that of East Africa – was due to the valuable resins from the frankincense and myrrh trees. In 450 BC, Herodotus, Greek writer and historian, extolled their virtues in quite lyrical form.

"The whole country is scented with them and exhales an odour marvellously sweet". The demand for frankincense and myrrh reached a peak about 2000 years ago when the caravans and their precious cargo, embarked on their journeys almost daily. Unfortunately, some of the myrrh was wasted during transport because the oil content easily escaped from the resin, unlike frankincense which was much more stable. Myrrh was pressed into goatskins to help retain the oil and frankincense was packed into basket-shaped containers to stop the 'tears' from sticking together. Although the resin trees grew plentifully in southern Arabia, the long arduous trek across the desert, packaging, labour and taxes meant that frankincense and myrrh became expensive commodities.

The route, it seems, began somewhere in the dry mountainous areas of the Yemen and Oman where the trees seemed to thrive on the limestone soil and intense heat – sometimes reaching 40 degrees centigrade in the shade. In his *Enquiry into plants, IX.3–iv 2*, Theophrastus mentions that "trees of frankincense and myrrh grew partly in the mountains, partly on private estates at the foot of the mountains; wherefore some are under cultivation, others not". Nevertheless, the Arabian traders were loath to reveal the exact location to the outside world – much to the chagrin of contemporary archaeologists who are still trying to determine the precise spot. It is reputed that these days the best frankincense grows in the Dhofar region in Oman, though Somalia and India provide other species.[8]

Until about 200 AD the caravans proceeded from their secret location and followed a westward route towards the Red Sea. Only the camel – charmingly referred to as 'the ship of the desert' – could survive the harsh vegetation and tortuous trail. A lighter breed of camel was preferred for desert conditions. The most ancient route – which was circa 2,400 miles long[9] is thought to have passed through Aden, Sana (capital of present day Yemen) and Tarim on to Sabota (now known as Shabway). It appears that there was only one main route at any one time because of the problem of arranging staging posts and ensuring security.

Many of the cities along the incense route prospered through taxes levied on the caravans. Sometimes the cities would take part of the resin in lieu of payment. Shabway was said to be the main inland trading centre. After the dues were paid the route continued through the desert of Seven Days, through to Marib, a large city which in 950 BC actually controlled the incense trade route. Marib was served by a great dam which irrigated the plain where the incense trees grew. The prosperity of the kingdom depended upon this dam for more than a thousand years. Marib was purported to be the domicile of the legendary Queen of Sheba (Saba). In 950 BC Sheba controlled the trade routes which transported the valuable commodities of those times: frankincense, myrrh, gold, ivory and an assortment of spices. Sheba was one of four countries that made up the spice kingdom. A powerful cartel developed controlling this giant industry which peaked in the second century AD, when 3,000 tons a year was shipped to Greece and Rome. Because the entire civilised world craved incense for their altars, the Spice Kingdom flourished from 1500–542 BC.

From Marib the caravans followed a close chain of wells at the eastern border of the mountains as far as Qarnawu. It then took a northward route following the Red Sea, along the winding coastal tracks and through the desert plains. Sandstorms, the piercing hot sun and marauding brigands turned the gruelling journey into a hazardous one. No wonder such a high price was put on commodities which put man and beast in such peril. 1200 miles and 90 days later, the precious cargo reached its destination. Assyria had controlled the northern end of the route until the 7th century BC. Shortly after, the Nabataeans, a tribe thought to originate from North West Arabia, began to control the export of resinous gums, balsams and spices to Europe. The centre of the 'sorting office' was the glorious city of Petra.

It was a magnificent city, carved out of huge rose and gold sandstone caves. For many centuries it profited as the main distributor for Arabia's incense and grew extremely wealthy. Its strategic geographic position placed it at the centre of the caravan cross-roads where six trade routes met[10]. Further, it was impervious to attack from rival tribes since it

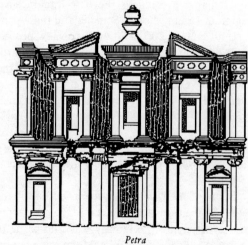

Petra

could only be entered through a narrow pass which was flanked each side by huge rock faces almost two miles long. Petra's dominance over the incense trade prospered under the Nabataeans. The merchandise was sorted and sent onward to the North Arab states and Syria, or west to Israel, Jerusalem, Egypt and the Roman Empire. The city became capital of an empire covering much of today's Syria, though it now lies in Southern Jordan, standing in magnificent ruin and visited by tourist and scholar alike.

These days, only a few hundred tons of frankincense are produced each year but during the time of Petra's sovereignty – around 300 BC – more than 3000 tons were exported annually. Interestingly, the most common artifacts excavated at the Petra site these days are the unguentaria – the ceramic receptacles used for incense, oils and ointments. The tapering bases of unguentaria vessels enabled them to be rested on the base of lamps thus releasing the aromatic vapours as the oil is warmed. Since a great number of the Nabataean unguentaria have been found in the Balkans and Europe, it is thought that they were also used to 'package' the oils and perfumes for export to the West.

Frankincense, as will be seen, has long been associated with the Sun god. The Nabataeans, it seems, worshipped the Sun with offerings of libations and frankincense *(Strabo XV1,4,26)*. The 'Temple of the Winged Lions' first built around 27 AD, actually dedicated to the fertility goddess Atargatis, contains an altar with a carved groove presumably for the placement of precious oils and incense. A carved grove on the floor of the 'Khasne' (The Treasury), the magnificent building at the entrance to Petra, suggests a place for animal sacrifice. The Nabataeans originally came from Arabia where incense offering was in fact a component of animal sacrifice.

Gaza became the main Mediterranean terminal for the incense trade in the first century AD. It was then transferred to Alexandria for sorting and sent to Greece and Rome. It seems that pilfering may have been rife at the sorting stations since Pliny wrote in his *Natural History (Bk 12, ch 32, sec 59)*: "At Alexandria ... where frankincense is worked up for sale no vigilance is sufficient to guard the factories. A seal is put upon the workmen's aprons, they have to wear a mask or a net with a close mesh on their heads, and before they are allowed to leave the premises they have to take off all their clothes".

Egypt

Trade between Egypt and Arabia was a lucrative one and rested primarily on frankincense and myrrh which the Egyptians used liberally in worship, medicine and perfumery.

It was said that the aroma of cedar and myrrh scented the Nile air. The Egyptians brought aromatics to a new level of expertise reaching a high point during the reign of the woman pharaoh, Hatshepsut c.1500 BC. Probably acting on the advice of her priests and physicians, Hatshepsut arranged for seedlings of frankincense and myrrh to be imported from the Land of Punt. It seems the Egyptians desired a home-grown variety. Punt was a country thought to be part of the southern Arab coast with Somalia opposite, though modern theory suggests Eritrea. There were many such expeditions but the tale of this one survives for posterity. It is chronicled on the walls of the spectacular temple at Deir el Bahri on the westbank of Thebes, present day Luxor. The Valley of the Kings lies just behind it, separated by high cliffs. The Punt reliefs record "… the loading of the ships very heavily with marvels of the country of Punt; all goodly fragrant woods of God's-land, heaps of myrrh resin, with fresh myrrh trees …"

The expedition probably set out from the harbour Leukos Limos (or Philoteras) on the Red Sea, then proceeded through the Gulf of Aden to the Indian ocean. They sailed along the African coast and anchored by Somalia or Zanzibar. Preserves, daggers, slaughtering axes and bright trinkets were traded for ivory, ebony, gold and 31 incense trees.[11] The artistic relief on the temple walls, deciphered by a professor Joannes Dumichen of Strasbourg informs us that the trees were planted in a huge garden in front of the temple.[12] The carvings remain but unfortunately, the trees perished. The Egyptians were expert gardeners and no doubt tended the young seedlings with the utmost care. However, it's possible that the variety brought back from Somalia might have been the 'coastal' type of tree which favour a rather more 'moist and salty' soil and climate. Some sources do say however, that myrrh trees were at some stage cultivated in Egypt.[13] If this is true, it would be a species of some very hardy variety.

NEFERTITI

Myrrh, like frankincense, had many uses. The beautiful **Nefertiti**, wife of the heretic Akhenaten (c.1570 BC) used an ointment containing myrrh. Her famous Bust, now in the State Museum Berlin, is certainly a testimony to her loveliness. When Akhenaten married Nefertiti, the couple received a wedding gift from the king of Mitanni consisting of two stone boxes containing myrrh resin and myrrh oil. Myrrh was an expensive gift in ancient Egypt. In one of the detailed Egyptian records from circa 2500 BC, it records that: "80,000 measures of Myrrh were being purchased by the pharaoh Sahure". We do not know what the individual measure represented in terms of weight, but clearly this huge volume must indicate how extensively myrrh was being used.

The unguent 'cones' shown on temple and tomb walls, were made from highly scented fat using plant materials such as sweet marjoram, myrrh, sweet flag and lotus. They were placed on the heads of male and female guests, and slowly melted from the heat of the head. The ointment ran down over the hair dripping on to the shoulders and gradually made its way over the upper part of the body.

Aromatics in the form of incense were mixed with perfumed woods like cedar and volatilised in glowing censers. Frankincense was used in 'censing' a god, a ritual which prepared the way for the performance of religious rites by a priest. It was burned in long handled censers by Priests stepping backwards in procession. In the New Kingdom, c.1550–1070, the censor had a kind of bronze baton topped by a falcon's head, at the base of which was a hand holding a small cup containing burning embers. The Priest brandished the censer in his left hand and with his right hand threw a pellet of incense into a cup[14]. Sometimes the offering of incense to the gods was performed by the king himself.

In the daily sacrificial rituals, the healing and intoxicating smoke apparently imbued the participants with religious ecstasy. The smoke was also a source of 'celestial food' for the gods, thought to be an insurance against 'evil spirits' who might send down pestilence and fevers to the populace.

Most important was the worship of the Sun God Re, symbolised as the Sun rising each morning on the eastern horizon in magnificent glory. It travelled across the blazing blue of the Egyptian sky, with its beams pouring down all day long, until commencing its journey through the night on the western horizon. To ensure the Sun God's return the following morning, incense was burned at the temple altar.

The offering of incense as a symbol of appeasement is depicted on a temple relief at Abu Simbel. King Ramesses II, c.925 BC, is shown plundering the temple of Jerusalem. High up on the ramparts is a figure offering an incense burner towards Ramesses asking forgiveness and mercy.[15] After the sacking of a city, it might be purified with frankincense. This was carried out apparently after the sacking of Memphis in the eighth century BC where the city was purified with incense and natron.

The Egyptian love of life was symbolised by their preoccupation with death. Convinced that the soul would at some future date repossess the body, death was believed to be a period of transition before eventual rebirth. Preserving the mortal remains therefore, became an important duty. It was well known that certain plants were able to preserve animal remains by inhibiting the bacteria which caused decomposition. The origin of Egyptian embalming dates back c.5200 years to the 1st Dynasty,[16] though a legend exists which attributes the actual rite of embalming to the goddess Isis. Apparently she reassembled the scattered body of her husband Osiris after it had been torn to shreds by his brother Set, and bestowed immortality upon him by anointing his body with precious oils.

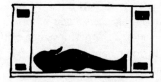 Traces of myrrh resin and rosemary have been found in the mummified bodies of Pharaohs, nobles and sacred animals, particularly at the site of the old capital Thebes (11th Dynasty 2133–1991 BC), present day Luxor. The west bank of Thebes, known as the City of the Dead, contained the tombs and housed the workers – carvers, quarrymen, draughtsmen – all those involved with the embalming process.

The practical business of embalming, which took several weeks to complete, began when the mourning period was over. The body was washed and the brain and viscera removed. Following the extraction of these organs, it was reported by ancient writers that the skull was rinsed with drugs including myrrh and the body cavity was packed with bruised myrrh. Following this, according to the *Bulaq Papyrus*, the head was anointed with frankincense. The body was then preserved in a salt-like substance called Natron after which it was further anointed with juniper, myrrh and cinnamon. Finally a variety of natural resins and Bitumen, (a black pitch-like substance referred to as 'Mum' – an Arabic word), were melted over a fire and poured over the mummy as a final seal.

Myrrh's use in the mummification process was to act as a preservative. The body of Menteptah, son of Ramesses II is an example of this. It was covered with fine linen which had been soaked in an aromatic yellow resin that dissolved in water (a characteristic of myrrh unlike other resins). Frankincense was seen as a precious gift to the gods. During the sacred work, the mortuary priests hired by the deceased's families, chanted solemnly in the background. The richer the family, the more priests hired and the louder the incantation. The priests wore masks featuring the jackal headed god

ANUBIS

Anubis, the god of embalming. Indeed, the ritual aspect was an important aspect of embalming and the burning of frankincense assisted in creating a sacred atmosphere. Its strong powers of evocation were thought to aid the souls of the departed rise heavenward in the smoke.

In 1922 the archaeologist Howard Carter, discovered the splendid tomb of Tutankhamen (1347–1339 BC) at Thebes. Amongst the artefacts were sealed unguent bottles, caskets and cool alabaster jars which revealed a hint of perfume after the seals were broken – quite astonishing after 32 centuries! The contents disclosed 90% animal fat and 10% resin.[17] Could they have been the legendary myrrh or frankincense? Their prolific use in the daily-life of ancient Egypt had ensured them a place in the after-life of the deceased.

The Holy Lands

There is evidence of incense being used in Syria and Palestine as far back as 2000 BC. Altars designed for incense burning have been found, one of which bore the Sun God symbol.

Aromatics in the form of incense were used by the Hebrews in significant amounts by 300 BC. Each morning and evening the High Priest burned the precious substance on the golden altar as prayers were offered up to God. Incense burning and the ceremonial use of flowers decorating the altar was a legacy of pagan rituals which continued throughout all the early civilisations. Among the many spices and resins used were cassia, spikenard, saffron, costus, mace, frankincense and myrrh. The earliest reference to aromatic substances is about 1,730 BC when the Ishmaelites came from Gilead with their camels bearing spicery, balm and myrrh, *Genesis 37:25*.

Writings in the 'Dead Sea Scrolls' advise all to take special measures on the Sabbath: 'Each person must launder their clothes and rub them with frankincense'. Every Sabbath day, shew-bread (holy bread) along with frankincense was presented on the table beside the altar in the Tabernacle. With other spices it was stored in a great chamber at the House of God at Jerusalem.[18] A special Biblical incense recipe for sacrifice was called 'Samin' and included four main ingredients: frankincense, myrrh, sweet flag and cassia.

Generally burning incense is thought to have been:

a) as a sacrifice to the deities
b) driving away evil spirits

c) sacrifice to a deceased person
d) symbol of honour to a living person
e) refreshing perfume at banquets and feasts.

When Moses returned from captivity, possibly in the reign of the Egyptian king Shoshenk 1, c 776 BC,[14] the inclusion of frankincense in Jewish observance was laid down in the Book of *Exodus 30:34.*

'Take unto thee sweet spices, stacte, and onycha, and galbanum; these sweet spices with pure Frankincense: of each shall there be a weight: And thou shalt make it a perfume, a confection after the art of the apothecary, tempered together, pure and holy:'

This blend was used to anoint the priests as well as all the religious trappings such as candlesticks and altars. 'Thy God hath anointed thee with the oil of gladness above thy fellows. All thy garments smell of myrrh and aloes, and cassia ... whereby they have made thee glad', *Psalms 45, 7–8.*

1 Chronicles 9:29 mentions that 'some of the sons of the priests made the ointment of the spices' and others were appointed to oversee the vessel, and all the instruments of the sanctuary, and the fine flour, and the wine, and the oil, and the frankincense, and the spices. Frankincense was often referred to as 'Lebonah' and afterwards renamed 'Olibanum' by the Romans.

The Old Testament tells us that pure and unmixed frankincense was the essential ingredient of the incense which was used at the temple[19]. The only place where frankincense should be used according to Jewish observance was in the worship of Yahweh, and any profanation of it was considered a capital crime deserving death.

Some thousand years before Christ, a meeting is purported to have taken place between the powerful and wealthy king Solomon and the fabulous Queen of Sheba. This is referred to in the Bible, in *1 Kings 10* and though there may be a kernel of truth in the fable, there is some doubt as to whether the kingdom of Sheba was really involved. If a ruling monarch from Arabia did visit Solomon, it might have been some head of the Sabaean tribe which controlled much of the incense trade.

The story goes that a romance ensued from this encounter, though the Queen's initial purpose for the trip to Jerusalem was solely an economic one. In the arid environment of her domain, spice and fruit fragrances were used widely and formed a considerable part of trade between Sheba and other nations. Spiced olive oil was employed as a cleansing agent and in body rubbing (massage). Myrrh and frankincense were used in purification ceremonies involving marriage.

Sheba (properly Saba) is an area believed to have been a country located on the southern edge of the South Arabian coast, almost opposite the horn of Africa. The Queen controlled the southern trade routes from India, Egypt and the horn of Africa. Trade was threatened when King Solomon's empire spread across the trade routes to Egypt. He controlled the northerly route from India and the west as well as to the Egyptian delta in the south and west to Damascus. Further, Solomon's Indian Ocean fleet of cedar ships was a large one and his vessels visited all the known ports. The artful Queen decided it was time to turn the tide against such fierce competition and resolved to visit Solomon in the city of Jerusalem *(I Kings 10:2)*.

This would have been a brave undertaking since the holy city was over 2000 miles away from Sheba. Nevertheless she travelled to Jerusalem, along with her large retinue, and legend has it that her beauty so dazzled the king that the trade routes were assured. However, the offering of spices, as well as frankincense and myrrh, probably helped seal the bargain. The marketable value of these resins can be discerned from the *Song of Solomon 3:6*. 'Who is this that cometh out of the wilderness like pillars of smoke perfumed with Myrrh and Frankincense with all the powders of the merchant?'

The seedlings the Queen left Solomon were apparently the foundation of orchards still in commercial use at the time of the suppression of the Jews by Titus Vespasian in 70 AD. Yet there was no evidence of the plantations when the Crusaders entered Palestine in the 11th century. Incidentally, it is reputed that Solomon planted his own seed in the Queen and a son was the result!

The most famous reference to frankincense and myrrh described in the scriptures is surely their presentation to the infant Jesus, along with gold. The three wise kings who offered these priceless gifts were thought to be Zoroastrian astrologer-priests from Babylon[20]. They had travelled to Bethlehem because the astrological conditions were right for the fulfilment of an Old Testament prophecy that spoke of the birth of a great leader *(Micah 5:2)*. A gift of the most highly revered articles of the ancient world was no doubt the greatest homage that could be paid to a king.

"When they saw the star, they rejoiced with exceeding great joy. And when they were come into the house, they saw a young child with Mary his mother, and fell down, and worshipped him: and when they had opened their treasures, they presented him with gifts; gold, and frankincense, and myrrh."

Matthew 2: 10 & 11

Christian tradition has it that these three kings come from South Arabia and it is possible that the three gifts consisted of the three spices, which are native of the Arabian Peninsula. These were frankincense, myrrh and balsam rather than gold, because a word spelt the same way as gold *dhb* served also to designate a kind of incense.[21]

The myrrh of the Bible is thought to be *Mecca balsam* produced from *V.* or *C. Opobalsamum* though the oft mentioned 'Stacte' in the Bible is believed to be another form of myrrh. Yet it is difficult to identify it nowadays. Myrrh is said to be one of the ingredients of the ointment used by Mary to anoint the feet of Jesus. Indeed, anointing the feet and garments of guests was a time-honoured custom. However, it appears that some objection was made to Mary's action by other people present. Jesus explained that she had anointed him for burial.

Myrrh was seen as a symbol of suffering and death by the Hebrews and was often used for anointing the dead. It was handed to Jesus on the cross mixed with wine, *Mark 15:23*. When the body of Jesus was taken down from the cross, Nicodemus used scented spices of myrrh and aloes to anoint Christ's body, since it was also a gum used for purification. Mary Magdalene and other women performed the last act for Jesus by embalming his body in white linen with herb and spices.

Many of the Christian martyrs were buried anointed with myrrh. The custom of burying with unguents and spices dated back to the earliest period of Christianity and may account for the divine odour so frequently reported upon when the tombs of saints were opened in following centuries.

The Christians, unlike the Greeks and Romans, did not believe that death was the end and a feeling of joy accompanied their last rites. Incense was burned at funeral processions and olive branches and palms were substituted for the mournful cypress. Christian funeral processions celebrated a victory not a defeat. When bodies of saints were transferred to more worthy resting places, their removal took the form of a procession consisting of chants and torches as well as incense and perfumes.

The church used incense for the forgiveness of sins whether the person was living or dead. This was carried out in a ceremony during which incense and prayers were offered up to God. Incense was also believed to have the capacity to restore a person to health by chasing away demons. This idea came from the early Chaldean and Babylonian belief that illness derived from some malevolent entity.

GREECE

The Greek preference for aromatics was influenced by a superb water supply, a very amenable climate and pleasant countryside. Orange, vine and olive trees encouraged more delicate floral fragrances. The Greeks were however, influenced by the ancient Egyptians' use of more exotic fragrances since Egyptian medicine and culture had long been an inspiration all over the East. It is estimated that at the time of Christ, around 3000 tons of frankincense was exported annually to Greece, as well as to Rome, from Southern Arabia.

Religion in Greece pervaded every aspect of personal and social behaviour. Altars were found everywhere; in secular public buildings, assembly places, temples, at the city gates and in the countryside at sacred places. The sacrificial offerings to the gods were initially of animal origin though incense took over around 400 BC. Yet in Homer's Odyssey, as far back as c.850 BC, reference is made to an incense altar in the temple of Aphrodite at Paphos, in Cyprus.

It is thought that the Greeks were influenced in the use of incense by travellers to Persia and Asia-Minor. Euripides c.400 BC speaks of 'Suria' – or was it Syria? – as the source of Frankincense. Sophocles c.400 BC was to write in his *Oedipus Tyrannus*: "Why sit ye here when all the city reek of the smoke of frankincense?". In Greek sacrificial ceremonies the incense was often carried by a virgin, on a flat circular basket on her head. The Greeks even included frankincense in one of their comedies. They had a scene where birds annoy the worshippers by preventing the frankincense smoke reaching the gods by dissipating it with their wings.

Much of our knowledge about the ancient use of incense derives from the writings of Greek philosophers and botanists like Theophrastus, who relates that frankincense was produced in the country of the Sabaeans, an active trading nation of antiquity, occupying the southern shores of Arabia. Plutarch reports that when Alexander the Great, the Macedonian-Greek general captured Gaza, 500 talents of frankincense and 100 talents of myrrh was taken and sent to Macedonia.

A Greek inscription of the third century BC on the ruins of the temple of Apollo at Miletus, records the gift made to the shrine by Seleucus II king of Syria (246–227 BC) and his brother Antiochus Hireax, king of Cilicia. This consisted of two vessels of gold and silver and ten talents of frankincense and one of myrrh.[22] Gifts of incense were a popular way of honouring friendship. Guests attending a banquet would have their beards perfumed with frankincense or the resin was burned on hot coals. There is some indication in Theophrastus that the Greeks may have burned myrrh on its own as an incense.

Rome

Shipping eventually superseded the camel as the chief means of transport and Petra which had been the central distribution point for incense, declined in prosperity. Much of the trade from southern Arabia to Egypt was subsequently carried along the Red Sea. Under the Roman Emperor Trajan (98–117 AD), Petra was absorbed into the Roman Empire. Roman looting became widespread and great quantities of incense was carried off from the city.

When Rome was at the height of her power, aromatics were used on a lavish scale, yet in 188 BC a Roman Edict actually forbade anyone to sell perfumed unguents and incense. All this changed of course. By around 23 AD it is estimated that a minimum of around 1300 to 1700 tons of frankincense was carried into the Roman Empire in some 7000 to 10,000 camel-loads annually. This amount was to increase in the following century.

The Roman Empire extended over southern Europe, Britain, Egypt and the Middle East. The Romans were adept at appropriating other people's ideas, and with their particular genius for organisation, they brought healing and perfumery to a fine art. Many of their ideas regarding hygiene, health and aromatics were of course, taken from the Greeks and Egyptians.

Aromatics were used to offset the stench of the dead beasts during the famous games performed in the arena. Large amphitheatres, like the Coliseum in Rome, were built to entertain the plebeians who were thought to like nothing better than to be subjected to endless amusement. Since the slaughter of man and beast often reached phenomenal proportions the stench of blood, increased by the hot sun, must have been quite pungent! Great braziers of incense were lit during the intervals and the aroma wafted over the grateful crowd. The Roman drainage system was quite spectacular with around 300,000 gallons of water pumped daily into the city from outside aqueducts. This enabled an elaborate sprinkler system to be constructed which turned on spraying fountains of perfume over the spectators.

Like other nations, the Romans also employed incense in worship. Frankincense, the most popular ingredient – alluded to as 'mascula thura' by Virgil – was sprinkled over hot coals on a small altar in the temples. Frankincense and myrrh were not however, confined to religious ceremonials. They were used on state occasions and in domestic life. 'My myrrh, my cinnamon' was a term of endearment. Plutarch even mentions that a statue of a bull made out of frankincense and other resins, was offered as a prize to the winner of a horse race!

The early Romans buried their dead but owing to Greek influence, bodies were cremated under a pile of scented woods and resins. At the funeral of important patricians (Roman nobility), vast quantities of incense and spices – chiefly frankincense and cinnamon – were laid on the pyres. The Emperor Nero (54–68 AD) and his wife Poppaea were enthusiastic users of perfume and cosmetics. According to Suetonius, Nero burned more incense at Poppaea's funeral than Arabia could produce in ten years! Unlike usual practice, Poppaea was not committed to the flames but embalmed after the manner of the Egyptians.

Pliny remarks on the huge amount of frankincense used in Rome, which was to increase substantially after his death. So much so that it may have contributed to the fall of the Roman economy since Rome was not a manufacturing country and its exports were small compared to its imports.

After Octavian (c.63 BC–14 AD) it was customary to deify the Roman Emperors. During the proceedings, incense was burnt in front of a statue of the reigning emperor as if he were already a god. In the reign of Justinian around 527 AD a 25% import duty was placed on luxuries, however, frankincense and black pepper were excluded as they were regarded as necessities.

The value of frankincense rested on its domestic and religious use, whereas myrrh was usually purchased by apothecaries for use in unguents, perfumes and medicines. There are some indications that myrrh was occasionally used in Roman cooking as a spice for appetisers. *(This may have some validity, because as myrrh is so bitter, a little in food will stimulate bile production preparing the digestive tract for the rich foods likely to follow.)* It was also added to wines to add a touch of astringency.

Pliny the Roman writer made a survey of the prices charged for commonly imported spices. The great interest in these figures is the indication it provided of the very extensive trading network to India and possibly even further.

	Denarii per pound
Frankincense best	6
2nd	5
3rd	3
Myrrh Stacte	3.5
Cave dweller	16.5
Erythraen	16
Scented	12
Cultivated	15
Cinnamon	300
Pepper, Black	4
Ginger	6
Nard	100

The cumulative price on a camel load of frankincense by the time it reached Rome was said to be 688 denarii. In Pliny's time between 1300 to 1700 tons of frankincense were imported to the Roman Empire. From this it was estimated that the total production in Arabia was around 2500–3000 tons per year. Over-cropping of the trees is known to have led to their extinction from many areas of Southern Arabia. This was compounded by the traditional use of the frankincense wood for cooking and camp fires.

Frankincense continued to be used in abundance in Rome right up to Emperor Constantine's time c. 312 AD. It is recorded in Vignoli's *Liber Pontifacalis*, Rome 1724–55, that Constantine presented the Bishop of Rome with costly vessels, fragrant drugs and spices as well as frankincense. Yet the use of frankincense dwindled sharply when the Romans turned to Christianity and banned pagan practices in the 4th century. There is doubt that the overland incense trade survived the fourth century and the sea-borne trade thrived only on a smaller scale. There was a revival of the incense route around the 6th century but demand for these valuable resins was not quite as extensive as in former times.

Modern Times

Marco Polo, that distinguished traveller, was one of the earliest visitors to Arabia after classical times. He reports seeing 'a large quantity of white frankincense of the best quality, which distils, drop by drop, from a certain small tree that resembles fir'.[23] Though frankincense continued to be looked upon with a kind of religious awe, its use in rituals declined around 622 AD after the rise of Islam. It was actually forbidden to be burned at funeral rites.[24]

Nevertheless old customs die hard. Travellers in southern Arabia, from the last century, describe how after the occurrence of death they witnessed recitations from the Qu'ran together with incensing with frankincense. This continued for three successive evenings between the time of prayer at sunset and the evening prayer. Furthermore frankincense was burned on the occasion when vows were made though it was not found among the spices which were used at wedding celebrations. Also the Yemenite Jews continued to burn copious amounts of frankincense at funerals. Fragrant spices of frankincense and basil were put between the folds of cloth in which the corpse was wrapped.[25]

Frankincense and myrrh are of course, still highly esteemed commodities in the Arabian peninsula, so much so that the scent of incense permeates everyday life in the Yemen and Oman. Incense burners are evident in public eating places and frankincense especially is a common ingredient of most households. In Oman it is customary to pass around an incense burner at the end of a meal where the men inhale and waft the fragrant smoke into their mustaches and beards. Receptacles are set up in front of mosques to receive the incense given by the visitors, and there is a Yemini satire in which a mosque complains that it has not obtained gifts of incense (buhur) for a long time.[26]

In the early part of this century, travellers visiting southern Arabia reported that the frankincense trees were owned by the Qara tribe but that they licensed other tribes to gather the incense in return for half of the crop's value. The coast of southern Arabia is visited by parties of Somalis, who pay the Arabs for the privilege of collecting frankincense.

The first scientific collection of specimens from Arabian frankincense was made in 1846 by Dr. H. J. Carter. He was surgeon in an East Indian company survey ship H.M.S. Palinurus surveying the south Arabian coast.[27] He first studied the branch of a species of frankincense tree thought to be similar to the Indian variety, B. serrata but later studies showed that it might be B. sacra. This was disputed and the tree origi-nally found by Carter was named after him B. carterii. However, it was later thought that the tree founded by Carter was probably of Somali origin. This is one example to illustrate how many varieties of frankin-cense trees exist and how difficult it is to distinguish between them.

Earlier this century a typical merchant wholesaled 20–30 tons of frankincense a year. For some time the commercial trading centre for incense gums has been Aden. Figures for 1913 show a trade of 140 tons of frankincense increasing to 250 in 1920 and 300 tons of frankincense and 70 tons of myrrh in 1975.[28]

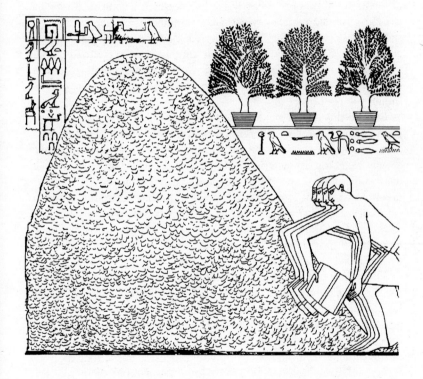

Botany and Habitat of Frankincense

Frankincense, or olibanum as it is known in the market place, belongs to the Burseraceae family. This family is further subdivided into many different species, approximately twelve of which belong to Boswellia, the Latin for the varieties which yield frankincense. Over 25 different species of Boswellia have been recorded. Numerous different varieties and sub-varieties have at one time or another been exploited for their oleo-gum-resin. Boswellia varieties grow throughout a wide geographical area ranging from East Africa to Saudi Arabia and across to the Indian sub-continent.

Even to this day there seems to be debate among botanists as to the precise identification of different types of frankincense and myrrh trees. This should not be surprising as it is common for wild plants to display a wide range of characteristics. This natural genetic diversity evolved over millions of years. Wide genetic diversity can make life hard for taxonomists trying to classify plants, and this inevitably leads to controversy. On the island of Socrata botanical expeditions have identified 6 species of Boswellia: *B. ameero*, *B. elongata*, *B. javanica*, *B. nana* and *B. popoviana*. This indicates how diverse the family is even over relatively small areas.

There are a number of writers who have claimed that the best quality frankincense only grows at elevations above 2000 feet, however clearly resin is produced from many areas. We also need to consider what is meant by quality; the assessment is frequently a subjective one and can depend to a large degree on cultural factors, or on the ultimate end use of the product. Even the ancient civilisations recognised that the yield from wild trees could be improved by transplanting them to other growing areas.

Some frankincense trees have been described as having finely cut deciduous (seasonal) leaves, white or pale rose flowers and pear-shaped fruits three-quarters of an inch long. Yet there are so many significantly different varieties of frankincense trees that it is extremely difficult to generalise on their appearance. Due to the differing types of this tree, and their varying chemical compositions, it can be seen that using specific botanical names for their essential oils can be highly misleading. The following are some of the different varieties which yield frankincense.

Boswellia carterii and *B. frereana* are native to the Red Sea region of north-east Africa, the major production areas are Ethiopia, Somalia and Oman.

Boswellia neglecta occurs in the Kenyan area and India.

Boswellia serrata is widespread and prolific in the Indian sub-continent.

Boswellia thurifera grows in Somalia, and is widely grown in India where a soft resin is extracted for incense.

Boswellia papyrifera is larger than other frankincense trees and grows in many places in Ethiopia, the Sudan and East Africa. The natives in Ethiopia claim that their tree was the true source of ancient frankincense but the truth seems to be that the resins were collected from an extremely large geographical area. Certainly the ancient writers were well aware of the various kinds of frankincense and myrrh trees.

Some frankincense trees in north east Africa and southern Arabia like to grow on rocky, soil-less hillsides whilst others prefer sheltered desert ravines. In Somalia however, some varieties grow mainly in valleys and the lower parts of hills inland and do not seem to like coastal air. Others hug the craggy coastal limestone cliffs.

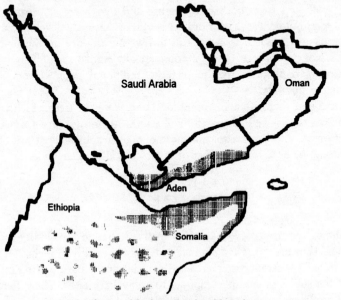

Principal areas of frankincense and myrrh production

SOMALIA

The Somalian tribes have names for several different types of Boswellia trees which are as follows:

Mohr meddu is the local name for the variety which yields *Luban Bedowi* or *beyo olibanum*. The tree is described as being 3–4 metres in height, with few branches. It is indigenous to the northern part of the country growing on limestone ranges at elevations up to around 1500 metres.

Maghrayt d'sheehaz is the name given to one coastal variety.

Murlo is the local name for the variety believed to be *Boswellia neglecta*. This tree attains a height of 5–6 metres, but the little resin which is obtained is mixed with other resins.

Yagaar is the name for *Boswellia frereana* and this yields the resin known as *Luban Meyeti*. This variety can grow up to 8 metres high and is often found clinging to rock faces by growing a bulbous base from which many fine roots penetrate deep into cracks in the rock.

The Arabian explorer of this century, Freyer Stark, found incense growing in the valleys of the Hadhramawt region. In 1949 an official report listed 11 ports from which frankincense was exported between Hadhramawt in the East and Quihn in the West.

Unfortunately, the Arabic name *luban* is often used to describe the resin collected from both frankincense and myrrh trees. Clearly the local terminology for the various types of trees has been developed over the millennia, and to this day still throws uncertainty on the precise sources of the various types of commercially traded resin. This is all part of the secrecy designed to keep the traditional income resource as hidden as possible.

Of course there are many other local names for the trees which yield frankincense as well as myrrh. The names obviously vary from one location to another across an enormous geographical area and one name can be used for a number of botanically dissimilar varieties.

OMAN

In Oman, the trees tend to grow in small scattered groups in dry rocky gullies. They are short and stunted with twisted thickly branching tops. A tattered appearance is created as the result of the bark peeling off in fine thin sheets in a similar manner to paper bark trees. The different grades of frankincense resin are identified by the traditional methods of smell, appearance and knowing the area where the trees are harvested. Over thousands of years the frankincense dealers at the ports have built up an enormous data base of traditional knowledge that is passed down the generations purely by word of mouth. This great expertise enables them (as with fine wines) to tell exactly where a particular batch of resin has originated and also if the payment due is reasonable for the quality of resin on offer.

INDIA

In India the main species is *B. serrata* with a number of different varieties. Known locally as *Salai*, this species is botanically and chemically quite different to its African cousins. The tree is particularly concentrated in the Vindhya and Satpura hills in Madhya Pradesh, the Aravalli hills in Rajasthan and Gujarat, and in central Andhra Pradesh. Collection of resin is not quite as widespread, being mainly concentrated in Rajasthan and Madhya Pradesh. The main use for these trees is for newsprint production. *Serrata* varieties are said to yield an average of 1kg of resin per tree. Once the resin has dried it is sorted into around 5 different grades with the long greenish coloured tears being considered the finest. Bombay is the main trading centre and a few years ago the yearly turnover was 800–1000 tons.

The *B. serrata* yields up to 16% of an essential oil upon steam distillation. It is pale yellow in colour, having a mild balsamic and pleasant smell. A mild camphoraceous note is characteristic of the Indian gum-resin. For the first two grades there is a good demand in the international market and they are almost entirely exported. The other grades are sold in the domestic market for consumption by the manufacturers of incense mixtures, oils and medicines. There is a good demand for ungraded material which is sold as a brown resinous product.

Some countries prefer the fragrance produced by *serrata* oils to that from *caterii* (and similar varieties) while others consider *serrata* inferior, but really such preferences are simply subjective judgments based on tradition. However it has been said that burning the whole resin in incense burners give a smell like 'burnt rubber'.

Currently there seem to be three major sources of frankincense: Eritrea, Somalia and India. However due to wars and droughts in the horn of Africa, major sources of supply can change quite quickly and can also result in the exploitation of varieties which are not normally traded.

Harvesting

Although the main source of oil is the bark exudate, in fact, the milky juice containing the volatile oil is distributed through the leaves and flowers as well as the bark. The leaves of some varieties are covered with glands containing an oil believed to be part of the tree's protection against overheating. This volatile oil is evaporated from the leaves by the sun's radiant heat, conducting away the heat thus cooling the vulnerable parts of the tree.

The resin is obtained from the bark either as a natural exudate or more commonly, by carefully scraping and chipping the bark away to reach the secretary ducts in which the milky white liquid resin is stored. This slowly oozes out forming soft beads which dry to yellowish 'tears' in the sun. These tears are then scraped off into baskets, the inferior quality resin that has run down the tree is collected separately. The cruder resins are often grey to whitish in colour and quite brittle. The crude resin has a balsamic fragrance and an aromatic, slightly bitter taste. If chewed it turns into a soft plastic mass.

In Oman harvesting occurs twice a year, in spring and autumn. This has to be carefully controlled as the trees can die if they lose too much moisture by over exploitation of the resin.

These trees have been a source of income for local tribes for thousands of years and therefore they do their utmost to protect the trees. The finest quality resin is said to come from the highland areas where during the gathering season the cutters camp out in local caves. Despite the widespread supplanting of camel power by jeeps in the Middle East, camels are still used to transport the resin from the remote gathering areas to coastal ports such as Aden, from where it is shipped all over the world.

The main fragrance use for frankincense is in incense burners. World-wide this consumes considerable amounts of the resin. The perfumery trade uses a variety of different grades of olibanum created by using different solvents and methods to purify the crude resins. These extracts are used as fixatives, for modifying the fresh notes of citrus colognes, for 'oriental type' perfumes and for men's fragrances.

Oleo-gum-resins possess many other properties useful to man and they have been used for numerous purposes. In India, quick drying timber varnishes are prepared from olibanum resin; also *B. glabra* resin was used for pitching the bottom of ships as it was particularly water resistant and once hardened, gave the wood some protection against marine wood borers.

Chemical Composition

The frankincense exudate or 'tears' consists of 60–70% resin, 27–35% gum and 5–7% essential oil, known in the trade as an oleo-gum-resin. Frankincense, therefore consists of three separate substances. The essential oil bound in the resin, should only dissolve in alcohol (or be separated from the resin by distillation). The gum portion should only dissolve in water. However in practice frankincense resin will fully dissolve in 90% ethyl alcohol as this contains just enough water to ensure almost complete solubility.

It is quite common for the commercially traded resins to be mixtures from different frankincense sub-varieties. Due to this, the chemical composition of essential oils extracted from the resin can be quite variable. Well over 200 different natural chemicals have been identified in various olibanum resins. Despite this chemical variation, most frankincense oils possess quite distinctive fragrances. Similarities in fragrance between different extracts despite wide fluctuations in the major chemical constituents are not uncommon. One reason is that the molecules which give an essential oil its characteristic fragrance frequently occur at levels as low as a few parts per billion. In other words it is only a tiny portion of the whole chemical make-up which gives the familiar aroma. These trace fragrance molecules are often so potent that they can overpower the 99.9999% of other natural chemicals in the oil, or they can blend with these other chemicals to produce 'synergistic' effects that give each extract (even from one crop to the next) a subtly different fragrance.

Another problem with attributing precise chemical compositions to frankincense resin extracts, is that it is common for wild growing plants to display huge variations in the chemical composition of their aromatic extracts. In the case of frankincense most extraction is from wild growing trees. Chemical variability is all part of natural genetic diversity which is frequently lost once plants are cultivated. It helps plants survive over millions of years as one disease will eliminate similar varieties, but others with slightly different genes will survive.

Once man starts cultivating plants, we can then obtain reliable extracts. An excellent example being Tea Tree oil. Most of this oil now comes from plantations where the cultivars used will always produce consistent quality essential oils with reasonably reliable therapeutic properties. Any oils produced from wild growing trees will be most unreliable due to the fact that one tree only a few metres away from its neighbour will have a totally different chemical profile. For fragrance purposes this chemical variability is not quite so important, however, for therapeutic use chemical composition can be critically important. For instance if frankincense is required for an anti-bacterial action, you simply cannot guarantee that it will work. This is because generally it would not be known if the molecules responsible for that action are in the oil used or not.

Some research using thin layer chromatography (a method of ascertaining the chemical make-up of any substance) has given promising results in being able to differentiate between the different botanical and geographical origins of Boswellia resins.[29]

In commerce, the oil from Eritrea is recognised by around 52% of octyl acetate*, whereas oil from Aden is recognised by the content of α-pinene being around 43%. In Somalia, the frankincense varieties of *Boswellia carterii* and *B. frereana* display the following compositional variation:[30]

B. carterii (Bejo)	B. frereana (Maidi)
α-thujene 19%	α-thujene 10%
α-pinene 7%	α-pinene 0.7%
Sabinene 9%	Sabinene 3%
p-cymene 3.5%	p-cymene 4%
limonene 8%	limonene 3.5%
β-caryophyllene 5%	β-caryophyllene 0.4%
α-muurolene 7%	α-muurolene 0.6%
caryophyllene oxide 3.5%	caryophyllene oxide 0.2%
unknown compounds 0.5%	unknown compounds 26%

West African Olibanum comes mainly from *Boswellia neglecta* and *Commiphora africana*. These varieties tend to be high in their α-pinene content averaging around 20–65% and the rest comprising small amounts of the chemicals common in other olibanum varieties.

Indian olibanum is mainly from *Boswellia serrata*. The resin yields up to 16% of essential oil. As with other boswellia varieties the chemical composition seems highly variable. Some researchers have found α–&–β pinene at high levels, others have found high levels of d-α-thujene and others high levels of d-limonene.

variety 1	variety 2
sabinene 60%	sabinene 5%
p-cymene 5%	p-cymene 4%
α-pinene 4%	α-pinene 8%
α-thujene 8%	α-thujene 61%[31]

Botany and Habitat
of Myrrh

The botany of the myrrh species is so complex that a whole book could be devoted to them. (Interestingly one variety has been named '*Commiphora confusa*'. Could this be the result of the great difficulty that botanists have experienced in the classification of the numerous different varieties?) Therefore here we will just present information on the trees which are *said* to yield the myrrh of commerce.

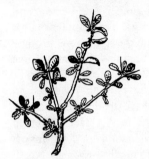

It is also difficult to attribute general characteristics to the trees which yield myrrh. For instance many have spines and thorns, but others do not. The flowers can range from whitish-green to yellow or red. The leaves are often trifoliate (3 lobed) but others are single. The best thing is to leave it to the botanists to argue about for another two hundred years.

The trees from which myrrh resins are harvested belong to a large genus of trees called *Commiphora*. Over two hundred and fifty species of Commiphora are recorded, many of which grow over a wide arc

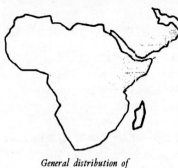

from Southern Africa to Arabia and across to India. Some varieties are widespread, whereas others only grow in very limited locations.

There are so many species of Commiphora that as recently as 1985 in a report in the Kew Bulletin, a botanical report had to be revised to include 'newly discovered species'.

General distribution of
Commiphora species

The species *Commiphora myrrha nees*, is described as having very spiny branches and twigs. The leaves grow in small tufts and consist of three leaflets up to 2 cm long. The flowers have short stalks and are white to light green, they produce a fruit 1 cm in diameter. Many people

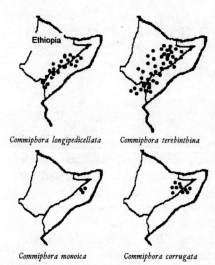

Commiphora longipedicellata   *Commiphora terebinthina*

Commiphora monoica   *Commiphora corrugata*

have described the tree as looking very similar to old European hawthorn bushes. Some are more like gnarled bushes of 2 metres high, while in other locations they can be more tree-like and up to 5 metres high.

The ancient authors such as Theophrastus and Pliny tried hard to find out about the botany and origin of frankincense and myrrh, but all their descriptions contain errors and anomalies. The main reason for this was that the Arabian tribes, on whose land the trees grew, strongly discouraged visitors because the trees represented their primary source of income.

A good deal of myrrh in Africa has always been produced in Somalia and Ethiopia. War and droughts have tended to shift the centres of production around over the years. In Arabia, the Yemen has always been an important centre for production. In 1920 myrrh trees were reported as being cultivated at Qu'tabah 100 miles North of Aden.

Myrrh resins are always in demand, and if the normal sources are not accessible, it is common for less commercially viable sources to be bought back into production. Such unreliable sourcing of material obviously leads to massive variations in the quality and in particular the chemical composition of myrrh resin.

Most resin is said to be collected from 'wild' trees, but as we know they can be cultivated, one must question how wild the trees really are. Many of them may have been planted by past generations of tribes' people who recognised their inherent worth for future generations.

Southern Arabian myrrh trees tend to be short (less than 3 metres) and highly branched, looking more like a bush than a tree. The bark is greyish-white and cracks naturally which allows the resin to seep out. The resin then hardens into masses which can vary in colour enormously from dark-yellow through to dark reddish-brown. The branches contain numerous long thorns.

Harvesting

The oleo-gum-resin fills natural fissures in the bark, or exudes following damage caused either by animals chewing the bark, or more commonly by incisions made in the bark in a similar manner to rubber tapping. The trees after tapping need 6 months to 2 years to recover. If because of easy profits, this time is not allowed, particularly if little rain falls, then the trees wither and die. It has been said that the trees appreciate the soil being raked around their bases as 'it cools their roots'. The oil is extracted from the resin by steam distillation, by chemical solvents including carbon dioxide, or by dissolving the resin in alcohol. The yield of oil is round 3–10%.

Description

In pharmacy the resin tends to be divided into two main types: Heerabol and Bisabol.

The Heerabol type is described as occurring in hard rough tears of 2.5–10 cm in diameter. The colour is usually reddish-brown and a fine powder covers the granules. Bisabol type is a deeper yellow and softer resin than Heerabol.

The oil can range from pale yellow to greenish or orange-brown, fairly thick and becoming sticky with age. Myrrh is one of the few essential oils whose fragrance improves with time, though it also becomes extremely gummy *(polymerised)* and almost impossible to pour. The fragrance is slightly spicy with characteristic incense-like notes. It has sharper pungent 'top notes' when fresh, these mellow and develop a 'warmer' character as the oil ages. The fragrance can vary a lot due to the numerous different tree varieties used for oil production.

Chemical Composition

The chemical composition of the different kinds of myrrh resins is very complex. Therefore we shall just give some of the more basic technical information.

There is a significant difference between the chemical composition of myrrh *resin* and the *essential oil* extracted from it. This is because many chemical compounds will only dissolve in water-based solvent (aqueous), while others are only dissolved in an oil-based solvent (lipid). Hot distilled essential oils will generally only contain high levels of the lipid soluble constituents, while alcoholic tinctures will contain water-soluble compounds as well as some lipid soluble compounds.

Myrrh resin correctly termed an 'oleo-gum-resin' is so called because the crude product contains a lipid soluble *essential oil*, a water soluble *gum*, and a *resin* which is soluble in alcohol. Myrrh resin comprises around 60% gum, 35% resin and only 5% essential oil but these figures can vary significantly.

The resin and gum portions contain numerous compounds which do not occur in the essential oil. This is critically important when specific therapeutic effects are required. For instance, it is no good expecting a mucous membrane astringent effect on the gums from the essential oil, if traditionally water or alcoholic extracts of the *whole resin* have been used. The essential oil may perhaps have superior anti-inflammatory properties, but its actions will certainly differ from extracts of whole myrrh resin.

The resin portion of the oleo-gum-resin may contain α-β-and γ-commiphoric acids, α-and β-heerabo-myrrhols, and many others. The *gum* portion will contain polysaccharides such as: arabinose galactose, xylose, also mucic acid, carbohydrates and proteins.

The composition of the *essential oils* as with the resin can be extremely variable due to the factors mentioned above. A complexity of sesquiterpenes is generally encountered.

Analysis of one sample of *oil* gave:

d-elemene	29%
copaene	10%
bourbonene	5%
β-elemene	6%
methyl isobutyl ketone	5.5%
2-methyl-5-isopropenylfuran	4.5%
plus many other sesquiterpenes in small amounts	

Analysis of 20 samples of C. africana *oil* from Kenya gave the range:

α-pinene	24–56%
β-pinene	4–12%
α-thujene	4–42%
sabinene	0–10%

para-cymene	0–28%
limonene	0–8%
terpinen-4-ol	0–13%
verbenone	0–7%
myrcene	0–2%
camphene	0–3%

A common feature of many of the different varieties is high levels of α- & β-pinene, some have high levels of sabinene and some high levels of α-thujene. Other analysts have reported: curzene 11.9%, furanoeudesma-1,3-diene 12.5%, 1,10 (15)-furanodien-6-one 1.2%, lindestrene 3.5%, curzererene 11.7%, plus many other unusual trace compounds.[32]

A Catalogue of some of the Burseraceae

(Myrrh & Frankincense)
Otherwise known as balsam trees due to
the presence of resin ducts in the bark

As can be seen, there are a great number of varieties – in fact there are too many to mention all of them here. These days more data is available about the varieties and grades of frankincense than is known about myrrh. Yet uncertainty still exists, since the information from different sources is often conflicting.

Myrrh (Commiphora)

C. africana
C. allophylla
C. baluensis
C. bruceae
C. ciliata
C. confusa
C. corrugata
C. dalzielii
C. danduensis
C. edminii
C. engleri
C. erythraea
C. foliacea
C. fulvotomentosa
C. gileadensis
C. guidottii
C. habessinica
C. horrida
C. kataf
C. lindensis
C. madagascarensis
C. myrrha
C. neglecta
C. oblongifolia
C. puguensis
C. quadricincta
C. rostrata
C. serrata
C. sphaerophylla
C. truncata
C. ugogensis
C. unilobata
C. velutina
C. virgata
C. zanzibarica

Frankincense (Boswellia)

B. brichettii
B. carterii
B. dalzielii
B. elongata
B. frereana
B. glabra
B. javanica
B. microphylla
B. nana
B. neglecta
B. ogadensis
B. papyrifera
B. popoviana
B. rivae
B. sacra
B. serrata
B. thurifera

Medicinal Uses of Frankincense – Ancient

'A garden enclosed is my sister, my spouse; a spring shut up,
a fountain sealed. Thy plants are an orchard of pomegranates, with pleasant
fruits; camphire with spikenard, spikenard and saffron; calamus and
cinnamon, with all trees of frankincense; myrrh
and aloes, with all the chief spices'.

Solomon 4: 12,13,14

In ancient times, only the pure in mind, body and spirit were allowed to commune with the Divine. The supplicant, prior to his union with the deity, was cleansed in body with myrrh and his spirit purified with frankincense.[33] The haunting aroma of frankincense may have endowed the proceedings with a mystical air but it was also a very efficient fumigant. Both in spiritual and secular practice, frankincense was either burned alone or with other odorous resins to banish disease carrying flies and mosquitoes. It was of course, employed in various medical preparations and its use seems to go back thousands of years.

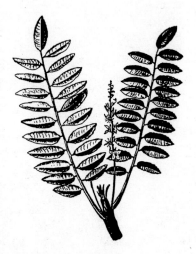

The many and varied medicinal uses are probably summed up in the 'Syriac Book of Medicine' which is based on a collection of lectures given by an unnamed doctor in Alexandria c. 4th or 5th century. It was used for nose-bleeding, headaches, ailments of the eyes and ears, gout, palsy, diarrhoea, ailments affecting the voice and the lungs, coughing, catarrh, pleurisy, stomach pains, diseases of the liver, kidney and bladder complaints, hardness of the spleen, nausea, ailments of the anus and dysentery.

Treatment for Wounds

Historically, frankincense has been widely accepted as an ideal treatment for various types of skin lesions; by implication this indicates possible antimicrobial activity. The ancient Egyptians certainly were well aware of its properties and used huge amounts in a wide variety of cosmetic and medicinal formulas. An Egyptian princess, suffering from an eye problem after using some new make-up was taken to see Imhotep, the grand priest, architect and physician who lived around c2630 BC. Inflamed eyes and ingrowing eyelashes were causing the princess great pain. Imhotep pulled out the eyelashes with tweezers, and after the eyes were cleaned, he massaged them with a cream of frankincense and other ingredients.[34]

There are some indications from ancient Egypt, that viscous resins such as frankincense may have been used as a form of sticky tape. This was mainly for holding the edges of wounds together long before stitching was developed.[35] Only in more modern times has it been rediscovered that it is better to hold wound edges together with strips if the wound is infected, rather than to use stitches which prevent the escape of pus.

Around 400 BC Hippocrates, known as the 'father of modern medicine', wrote a prescription for obstinate ulcers. This prescription contained the metallic compounds commonly used at that time, as well as frankincense, myrrh, gallnuts and vine flowers. The metal salts would have been antibacterial and slightly astringent; the myrrh and frankincense possibly provided a pleasant perfume to a malodorous wound as well as contributing their mild antimicrobial, drying and healing effects. The gallnuts and vine flowers are powerful astringents drawing together the open wounds. It was common in ancient Greece to include some frankincense in salves made for treating sores and wounds.

 In Arabia broken limbs were treated with the soft gum placed between layers of bark. This was then tied around the broken leg or arm and as the resin set it formed a perfect mould to the shape of the limb, similar to a modern plaster cast.[36]

Other civilisations have also found frankincense to be very effective on skin complaints. For instance, in China, it was the constituent of several skin remedies, including those for bruises or infected sores. It was also used for wounds in India as well as being a remedy for rheumatism. In Kenya it was used to treat wounds, and blood in the urine resulting from schistosomiasis. This is a parasitic infection of the blood; the parasite enters the skin from contaminated water which is common in African countries.

URINARY, REPRODUCTIVE AND RESPIRATORY SYSTEMS

In some eastern countries the bark of frankincense was boiled in large quantities to make a wash for fever and for internal usage for gastro-intestinal troubles. A decoction of the root boiled and taken in copious draughts was used as a remedy for syphilis. Both the bark and root were boiled as an antidote to arrow poison. The mixture was taken internally, and after a few hours it was said to relieve the symptoms of giddiness and palpitations.[37]

β-boswellic acid in the oleo-gum-resin has been reported to display anti-inflammatory and analgesic activity.[38] Now we know that β-boswellic acid has been found to display anti-inflammatory and analgesic properties, this perhaps gives justification for the use of frankincense for urinary tract infections.

Al-Kindi, an Arab physician of around 850 AD wrote a 'Medical Formulary' which included at least 6 prescriptions containing frankincense (see Formulas). Avicenna the Arab physician of the 11th century refers to frankincense for inflammation and infections of the urinary tract. He also advocated it for tumours, fevers, vomiting, and dysentery. Also in Arabia, according to Pliny, frankincense was used as an antidote to poisoning.

Frankincense was often combined with myrrh in treatments for medical problems. Celsus suggested that the following ailments would respond to their healing powers: relief of pain in the side and of liver problems, inflammation of the ears and eyes, haemorrhoids, bladder-stones, inflammation of the vulva and genitals, for inducing menstru-ation and for 'broken-heads'.

The red underbark, as well as making a dye, was also chewed in pregnancy to alleviate morning sickness.[39] Jewish Yemenite women used to kindle frankincense (lebona) beneath a wife in labour so that the smoke entering her body would enable her to deliver the child with ease.[40] On the third day after childbirth, the women assembled for a celebration and burned frankincense. Each woman stood for a while over the incense burner for incensations. This was particularly beneficial for the 'mother' as frankincense was believed to heal birth scarring and reduce post-natal infections.[41] It was customary for a woman to stay in the house for 40 days after childbirth. When she left the house for the first time she was incensed with frankincense.

The National Dispensatory, A Stille & J. M. Maisha 1879 suggests its use in expelling lochia (vaginal discharge of mucous and blood following childbirth), as well as promoting menstruation and as an ingredient for the treatment of leucorrhoea. It was also said to be useful as an expectorant in bronchial catarrh and infantile asthma. It was applied in ointments for various ulcers, including those caused by burns as well as chilblains, cutaneous eruptions and inflammation of the eyes. More recently it was an ingredient of various stimulating plasters and its fragrant fumes used to counter unpleasant smells.

Other uses

The gum was employed in early forms of dentistry. In Arabia pieces of it were chewed, mixed with salt and then used to plug holes in teeth. The fresh gum was also applied as a hair lacquer. When dried this would hold in place elaborate hair styles. Indian doctors recommended the use of the resin, mixed with clarified butter 'for gonorrhoea and the bloody flux'.

The leaves of the frankincense tree were used for animal fodder. Resin gatherers sold sacks of leaves to camel trains. They were considered the finest remedy against diarrhoea in animals. In times of famine, the Khnoods and Woodia tribes in India live on a soup made from the *B. serrata* variety.[42]

John Gerard, writing in his *Herbal* (1633) tells us that frankincense 'filleth hollow ulcers and close raw wounds' indicating its continued use for skin lesions. He also quotes the Greek doctor Galen who said that '*it heats in the second degree and dries in the first*'. Culpeper (1616–1654) explains the meaning of this in his Herbal. Under 'Temperaments of the Herbs' he says that all medicinal plants were considered either *hot, cold, moist, dry or temperate* in respect to man's own bodily heat. Each 'plant temperature' was graded in degrees from 1 ascending to a powerful 4. Those plants for instance that were hot in the first degree were in equal temperature with our bodies and restored warmth if the body were cooled by disease or accident. Frankincense being hot in the 2nd degree would 'by outward application abate inflammations and fevers by opening the pores and taking away obstructions'. The 'drying' medical plants had the effect of reducing phlegm and excess mucous and moisture in the body. Drying in the 1st degree was 'strengthening'.

It is interesting that *Redwood's Pharmacopoeia, Theophilus Redwood, 1857* reports that 'the gum resin olibanum and Indian olibanum is stimulant, astringent and diaphoretic (inducing perspiration)'. Different words used to express the same heating, binding and moisture curbing properties used by the 17th century apothecaries who had borrowed from the Greeks.

Medicinal Uses of
Frankincense – Modern

'The name of God be on you and myrrh and frankincense
and copal-resin and juniper-resin'

The above words were said as a form of blessing by women visiting a mother immediately after childbirth. This was an Arabic custom still prevalent at the beginning of the century[43] and in Dhofar a woman after bearing a child will still fumigate with incense.[44] Some women in Aden put frankincense on the fire and swing their child in the smoke, after first rubbing it with oil.[45]

These examples show that the protective power of incense, as well as its remedial effects, prevail to this day. In southern Arabia rooms are fumigated every day five or six times! This custom is also applied to the hair though perhaps not so frequently. The purpose is to remove flies and mosquitoes and the variety of frankincense used is said to be Boswellia Roxb.[46] In Sana the custom has survived of turning jugs upside down over burning frankincense after which they are filled with water. The water is imbued with the taste of frankincense and this beverage is drunk while chewing a stimulating herb called qat.

Until the early 1940's, a potion was prepared with pounded frankincense and dispensed as a drug against inflammation of the urethra, against phthisis (T.B.) and shock paralysis.[47] The girls from the tribe of the Qara in the mountains of Dhofar use a type of wax made of frankincense to remove pubic and axillary hair.[48]

An infusion of the bark is commonly mixed with an extract of pods of *Acacia arabica* and used in hardening and preserving the corpse amongst some Nigerian tribes.[49]

Male/Female

Apparently because of its bitter aromatic taste, larger and softer pieces of the resin are chewed by children and women – the latter especially in pregnancy. The pieces which are used for this are called *luban unta (female frankincense)* or *luban la (chewing frankincense)* in contrast to *luban dakar*, the *male frankincense*. The difference is said to be due to some resin exuding from the bark, which forms masses resembling testicles and so is classified as 'male'. This is much more expensive than those resins which form small 'tears' and is classified as the 'female' variety. Though tradition dictates that there is a difference between the two types, in practice, because of the softness of the resin when fresh, it is easily moulded into whatever shape pushes the price up.

A cure for arthritis?

Chinese herbalists use frankincense in a powder form and in teas for menstrual pain, and externally as a wash for sores and bruises. Besides helping to calm and clear the mind, frankincense is thought to be highly antiseptic. It was used for leprosy, cancer and pulmonary tuberculosis and in teas for rheumatism. Indeed the alcoholic extract of the defatted gum resin has shown marked anti-arthritic activities.[50] The steam distilled essential oil from *C. caterii* with 60% l-octyl acetate was found to inhibit the growth of a number of pathogenic bacteria. It was noted that the hexane extracted essential oil, did not have anything like as potent antimicrobial activity.[51]

Resin obtained from *Boswellia serrata* (local name *salai gugal*) has been used in traditional medicine in India for treating chronic inflammatory arthritis. Some of the resin's constituents called boswellic acids have been tested. In trials on isolated tissues these compounds were found to have an anti-inflammatory effect. Of particular interest was the report that boswellic acids seem to have a very low toxicity.[52]

Nervous diseases

A report on *Boswellia serrata*[53] seems to confirm the use of frankincense upon the emotions. It was reported that it was widely distributed in the central and western parts of Arabia and the gum resin obtained from it is used in the treatment of many nervous diseases. The resin is still taken in Arabia to dispel forgetfulness, to treat various type of psychological disorders and to dispel lethargy.[54] It would seem that scientific investigations of the numerous chemical compounds occurring in plant extracts, together with a greater understanding of how fragrances are perceived by the brain, means at long last we are beginning to realise that some of the ancient uses for frankincense have a very sound foundation. The widespread and timeless use of frankincense in religious worship would never have persisted for so long if it did not have recognisable effects. Religions are obviously aware that frankincense in particular can have an effect on the mind conducive to meditation and prayer.

The use of aromatic materials from plants is playing an ever increasing role in treating various kinds of stress related disorders. There is an increasing body of evidence to suggest that mental stress has a depressing effect on the immune system, but equally, the use of pleasing aromas may be beneficial. If one can relax in a room filled with a beautiful fragrance, have a relaxing fragrant massage, or unwind in a perfumed bath, then emotional stresses can be eased. Certainly many people agree that frankincense has emotionally uplifting and soothing effects.

Effective decongestants

While extensive use was made of many essential oils by the medical profession between 1800 and 1900, frankincense oil seems not to have gained recognition when the major national pharmacopoeias were being produced. Considering how extensively it had been used in ancient times this seemed incredible. Though several mentions were made about the use of the *powder* in 'fumigating mixtures'. *The National Dispensatory 1879* describes the uses attributed to frankincense by Hippocrates, i.e. to promote menstruation, ointment for ulcers and burns, for chilblains and eruptions, as expectorant and for asthma. Earlier the Egyptians had used frankincense to treat coughs and asthma.

Both the resin and the oil are effective expectorants and decongestants, and the vapours of frankincense are ideal for diffusing in the rooms of people suffering from bronchial congestion. The essential oil used in room diffusers is particularly beneficial for anyone suffering from irritating night cough or bronchial complaints that disturb sleep. The relaxing fragrance may help soothe the mind as well as the throat, thus ensuring more peaceful sleep.

Five cases of therapy with frankincense and myrrh were documented in Jamaica and London involving the respiratory system. In Jamaica, a two year old child was admitted to hospital with severe malnutrition, a cough with respiratory distress and poor appetite. Treatment consisted of antibiotics and a nutritional regime while the mother also insisted on the use of an oral remedy containing frankincense and myrrh. The child steadily recovered and was discharged well-nourished 6 weeks later.[55] In London, a three year old child was admitted to hospital because of respiratory distress with a fever, dry cough, vomiting and anorexia. The orthodox treatment incorporated antibiotics and intravenous fluids though the father was allowed to give his son a medication consisting of fine granules of frankincense and myrrh mainly intended as a cough remedy. The child was discharged 7 days later and his clinical signs resolved over 6 weeks.

However, it is crucial to differentiate between the use of frankincense as a fragrance and its use as a medicinal substance via the gastro-intestinal tract. The latter use needs professional guidance from a medical herbalist or other traditional healer. The physical healing effects on the body achieved by the internal uses of water or alcoholic extracts of frankincense and myrrh resins, will almost certainly differ from the effects of using their essential oils. A pure essential oil contains a significantly different range of substances from the traditional water or alcoholic extract. It must be emphasised here that there is very little traditional use of the *essential oils* of frankincense or myrrh. Therefore, these essential oils must not be taken as medicines internally.

USES OF FRANKINCENSE IN AROMATHERAPY

Many aromatherapists choose frankincense in blends which help to alleviate stress and aid relaxation. But there are many sedative-type oils; why should frankincense be chosen instead of other equally effective oils? Naturally, the choice of essential oil depends upon the client/patient. The relaxing effect of frankincense is very helpful perhaps when the person feels confused or reaching a difficult crossroads in their life. Like its ancient use in worship, frankincense can help restore faith and equilibrium into a person's life. Used in massage, perhaps combined with lavender and geranium, it can be a balancing and soothing blend.

Frankincense can also be used for cold symptoms, particularly where there is difficulty in breathing and possibly in cases of asthma, influenza, bronchitis, sinusitis and catarrh. As a *room-fragrance* frankincense combines well with cinnamon leaf and ginger – the vapours will help to clear the lungs and break-up mucous. The smell of this blend can have distinct effects on the mind and emotions. Some people find it relaxing while others feel invigorated. As a chest *rub* for any of the above respiratory problems, substitute the cinnamon leaf for lavandin, rosemary or sandalwood, depending on the person and the circumstances. The unrefined resin or the pure essential oil can be added to hot water for inhalation of the vapours in cases of bronchitis, laryngitis and coughs. For an effective expectorant and decongestant, add 3–4 drops of the oil, or a teaspoon of the resin.

The Egyptians used frankincense in many of their face-rejuvenating ointments for its pleasant fragrance and possibly as an aid to the preservation of the ointment. For dry skin frankincense is often combined with rose and chamomile in·a non-perfumed *cream* and for greasy skin, frankincense is said to blend well with bergamot and cedarwood. Frankincense may also be added in small amounts to the *bath* to provide a very relaxing and tension relieving environment which will also help treat damaged skin or any sore, irritating ailments. For this purpose however, it should not be used more than once or twice weekly. Care should also be taken that adverse skin reactions do not occur due to pre-existing allergic conditions.

Some aromatherapists use frankincense with either bergamot, sandalwood or juniper to combat problems of the urinary tract such as cystitis. However, whether this actually works on the psychological or physical level is speculative.

For an exotic room fragrance, combine it with galbanum, geranium and orange.

Medicinal Uses of
Myrrh – Ancient

"And let the king, my Lord, send troops to his servants
and let the king, my Lord send Myrrh for medicine"
Letter sent to Amenophis IV from Palestine c 1370 BC
(then part of the Egyptian Empire)

Gums, resins and plants have been used as medicines since the very early civilisations. In reviewing the historical uses of myrrh particularly, it would seem that it was generally looked upon as a 'cure-all', especially in the east.

Assyrian cuneiform texts give us a broad view of the number of ailments for which it was employed in Mesopotamia. It was a constituent of poultices for the head and utilised in treating chilblains and ailments of the eye, ear, nose and anus. It was also mixed with alum for a mouthwash, prescribed for strangury (difficulty in voiding urine) and applied as an enema. Solutions of myrrh resin were used for mouth infections and as a medium for other drugs. In Assyria myrrh was burned in a censer, which was placed at the head of a sick person's bed, possibly acting as a fumigant. It was also used in this way for clearing blocked nasal passages, headache, vertigo and cloudiness of the eye.

In the Syriac 'Book of Medicine' myrrh features in a large number of prescriptions for a wide variety of ailments, frequently in conjunction with frankincense. These were for headache, delirium, falling sickness (epilepsy), paralysis, fatigue, palsy, gout, coughs, constipation and dysentery.

Sumerian medical texts, c.1700 BC, contain a number of recipes with myrrh as a constituent. The mention of 'essence of cedar' in these same recipes is fascinating as it strongly indicates the Sumerians had a knowledge of some form of distillation. Indeed Sumerian pottery vessels capable of a crude form of distillation have been found and dated to around 3500 BC. This important archaeological find indicates that distillation may have been used to produce medicines and perfumes by some very ancient civilisations.[56]

Wounds

Myrrh was much in demand for the healing of wounds and appears to have been valued as a disinfectant. Moreover, it seems to have been useful for its 'binding effect'. The wound was cleaned and then smeared with myrrh which apparently secured the surrounding tissue. Assyrian medical literature reveals that myrrh and other resins were common ingredients of 'wound remedies' used possibly for their mild antibiotic properties as well as to fumigate malodorous wounds.

Myrrh appeared well identified in many Egyptian prescriptions named *antyw*. It was formed into plasters with honey and then used externally for various types of wounds. This type of preparation would provide a mild, but effective, antibacterial action. An Egyptian recipe for 'a wound in the neck' was: myrrh one part, with four of the djpt plant. This was worked into a mass and bound on to the neck.

Around 400 BC Hippocrates wrote a prescription for obstinate ulcers and Theophrastus c. 370 BC used a formula containing myrrh, burnt resin, cassia and cinnamon to treat inflamed wounds. The Romans dissolved lumps of myrrh resin in wine and applied this lotion in treating burns. It is also known that wine was used to wash wounds. There are some natural pigments in wine with proven antibacterial action, the addition of myrrh resin would have produced a highly effective lotion for treating all manner of wounds.

Sometimes called *mo yao* in China (though this name may be unreliable) myrrh has been used here since the 7th century, primarily as a wound herb and as a blood stimulant. It was also employed in treating conditions such as bleeding haemorrhoids, menstrual difficulties, sores, painful swellings and tumours as well as arthritic pain.[57]

John Gerard's Herbal 1597 extols the virtues of myrrh with regard to wounds ... "the marvellous effects that it worketh in newe and green wounds, were heere to long to set down".

The Head – mouth, ear, nose and eyes

Myrrh's reputation for oral hygiene is also well documented. In Mesopotamia it was mixed with alum for a mouthwash and to strengthen spongy gums. The Assyrians employed a popular lip salve of arsenic and myrrh. It was also used to check excess salivation and tonsillitis. During the 18th century, myrrh was added to preparations such as *electuaries* in order to treat the sore, rotting gums caused by scurvy in mariners. Many medications had been used for scurvy which included myrrh before it was known that vitamin C deficiency was the prime cause of the disease. Arab physicians recommended it for gum problems and suggested sucking on the resin.

Poultices including myrrh were also used for ear and eye inflammations as well as for nasal congestion. Culpeper mentions that the 'root of the yellow Daffodil boiled with honey, wine, myrrh and frankincense dropped in the ears, is good against all the corrupt filth and running matter in these parts'. Not that this is recommended! In any case, daffodil bulbs are poisonous.

Respiratory tract

Myrrh also seems to have been instrumental in helping pulmonary problems. The dust storms from the Sahara desert meant that the Egyptians would daily breathe the sand into their mouths and lungs, resulting in chest infections, blocked sinuses and headaches.[58] Myrrh was apparently helpful for diseases which affected the respiratory system, such as pulmonary tuberculosis, and was valued for its astringent, antiseptic, tonic, healing and stimulating properties. Indeed the Syriac book of medicine mentions that myrrh was used for most ailments of the respiratory, gastro intestinal and urinary tracts. Culpeper endorses its tonic and healing properties and recommends it for 'roughness of the throat and windpipe'.

Reproductive tract

The Arabs used myrrh for uterine ailments, 'flaccidity of the womb' and barrenness.[59] Its stimulant and tonic effects were said to be helpful for the treatment of amenorrhea (when it was often combined with aloes and iron). It was said to move stagnant blood through the uterus and to be helpful for the menopause, menstrual irregularities and even uterine tumours.

In the *Papyrus Ebers* c.1500 BC a medication for rectal prolapse is described as follows: 'For a displacement of the back part: myrrh, incense, reed nut from the garden, *mhtt* from the river bank, celery, coriander, oil and salt are cooked together, placed on cotton and put in the rear end'. In Mesopotamia myrrh was used in making poultices for wounds to the anal sphincter.

Other uses

Later Arab physicians were very much more selective in prescribing myrrh. They did use it internally for expelling intestinal worms. Al-Kindi, an Arab physician of around 850 AD, wrote a 'medical formulary' containing at least 15 different prescriptions using myrrh for a wide variety of conditions. The Arabs also used myrrh applied as a plaster for scorpion stings and as an antidote to the bites of vipers. The intense heat in Egypt and other eastern countries encouraged flies and insects which spread infection from dirt and rubbish to humans. Myrrh was made into pellets to rid the home of these disease-carrying insects. Celsus mentions that it was an ingredient in prescriptions and was taken internally. Besides being an antidote to poison, it was also used to cure dropsy, fever, relieve pain in the side and liver, for treating haemorrhoids, for genital inflammation and for abscesses.

Myrrh was a popular medication in Greece and Rome. It was used as an enema, and for inflammation of the ears, bladder-stones, inflammation of the vulva and genitals as well as in plasters for 'broken heads'. In many of these prescriptions it was compounded with frankincense. The Romans used myrrh and other aromatic materials boiled in water and added it to wine – they thought it would diminish drunkenness!

Though myrrh was included in the 'holy ointment' *(Exodus 30:23-24)*, many of the other supposed uses quoted in the Bible are open to question. Several different types of gum resins were commonly used in antiquity, and trying to work out which ones the translators of the biblical texts are referring to is extremely difficult.

Medicinal Uses of
Myrrh — Modern

"The Sultan sent to our camp some bowls of good
soup and a fowl cut up and cooked in gravey, very rich
with oil and onions. It would have been good but
for the bitter taste of myrrh, which they
like so much to put in their food"
A journey to the west of Aden

The power of fragrance to effect dramatic changes in physiological
function has been documented since ancient times. Traditional healers
have used the smoke from aromatic plants for thousands of years as a
critical part of healing rituals. We all know how the smell of food
triggers our digestive processes, or how other smells can make you feel
sick.

There is now a good deal of evidence to suggest that fragrance alone
can initiate indirect physiological changes via its effect on the chemical
pathways of the brain. Clinical trials have indicated that fragrance can
produce profound alterations in the immune system.[60] Such effects have
been well known since ancient times by traditional healers, but few in
the medical world would believe such 'superstitious nonsense'.

Myrrh is still very much part of traditional medicine in its production
areas. The uses it is put to vary somewhat depending on geographical
location and on the type of myrrh available. In the late 1800's the Arabs
were said to have burned the wood as fumigants to help nasal catarrh,
sciatica, vertigo, headache and cloudiness in the eye. In Somalia
depending on the location and variety, it is used in husbandry to
improve the yield of milking camels and in various venereal diseases.
While in other parts of Africa it is used as a fumigant to keep insects
away, as well as other numerous medicinal purposes.

Resin from *Commiphora guidotti* is used to treat stomach ailments
and diarrhoea. It must be emphasised how serious diarrhoea is in
underdeveloped countries. In Africa surveys have concluded that up to
50% of childhood deaths are due to this problem. Therefore any herbal
remedy that can help relieve the problem is of great value. In a survey

of Somalian medicinal plants *Commiphora multifoliolata* was found to be used for treating cholera.[61]

These days myrrh, the variety known as *qataf* (or kataf) is used in Somalia as a liniment for washing hair – that known as qafal is used as a purgative for horses. In Somalia today women who have just given birth, burn the wood of one species of myrrh to fumigate the house. It has also been given in a diluted emulsion to newly born children. The resin from another variety is used to treat stomach complaints, diarrhoea and to treat wounds. Some authors report that myrrh has been, and may still be used to treat the wounds caused by the barbaric practice of female circumcision. Myrrh from Somalia is imported into India and China. As recently as 1991 in both countries, it was said to be added to the food of cows and buffaloes to increase the quality and quantity of their milk.

Due to the different varieties of trees used to produce myrrh, its physical properties can however, be somewhat unreliable. Also the confusion with *bdellium* makes it difficult to determine the uses of the many varieties of myrrh very precisely.

Wounds

Myrrh is, of course, renowned for its use in wound healing preparations though it may well be that certain varieties are more efficacious than others. Whichever variety was used, it seemed to cause few side-effects, unlike many of the other more corrosive or poisonous preparations commonly used in those days. It seems myrrh is used for its antiseptic properties.

An important feature of the use of aromatic plant extracts to treat wounds is the psychological effect. Dirty wounds can smell very bad, if the aromatic material did nothing other than impart a pleasant odour, then the effects on the emotions of the patient would be substantial. Such uplifting effects on the spirits would very likely improve the immune status and enhance the healing process. Modern research is only just beginning to rediscover how important our sense of smell is to our well being and immune status.

Yet the direct application of myrrh has given some positive results. Three kinds of myrrh resin dissolved in water acted as effective antibacterial agents. They inhibited gram positive bacteria and inhibited the growth of *Staphylococcus aureus*.[62] This type of organism is especially responsible for the formation of pus as well as boils and carbuncles.

Also, anti-inflammatory activity was reported in individual natural chemicals found in *Commiphora mukul*.[63]

Screening of the resin of *C. rostrata* and its three major components showed considerable antifungal activity against Asperigillus and Penicillin species. It also prevented the growth of mycotoxins (the very dangerous poisons produced in contaminated food).[64]

The resin and tincture of myrrh have been used to treat leg ulcers but for this purpose the essential oil is much to be preferred. Myrrh oil diluted in refined coconut oil can be applied to leg ulcers or other poorly healing ulcers or wounds. It must be remembered that a herbal tincture made using water and alcohol, will not produce exactly the same therapeutic action as does the essential oil from the same plant. Water soluble therapeutic substances are generally dramatically reduced or entirely missing from distilled essential oils.

Oral Hygiene

Many herbalists recommend tincture of myrrh as an astringent for the mucous membranes of the mouth and throat.

Myrrh's use as a remedy for mouth ulcers and gargles for sore inflamed throat conditions has been used right up to modern times. It has even been included as an active ingredient in toothpaste. Tincture of myrrh is used for mouth washes, gargles, ulcerated throat, chapped lips and spongy gums. Myrrh itself gives a biting-burning, somewhat acrid-aromatic taste for mouthwashes however, in a tincture which is made by dissolving the crude resin in alcohol. The tincture has been considered by many to be the remedy of choice for mouth and gum ulceration, for spongy and unhealthy gums as well as for throat infections. It is effective treatment for pyorrhoea and gingivitis, a common infection of the surface tissue of the gums.

Mrs. C. Leyel a prolific writer on herbal remedies in the 1930's to 50's said: "As mouth washes and tooth powders, it is one of the most useful antiseptic applications for the gums and mucous membranes. For spongy and unhealthy gums, it can hardly be equalled as it is astringent as well as healing." She goes on to say that "taken internally its stimulating action diminishes excessive secretions from mucous surface, quickens the cardiac action, acts as a gastric stimulant and tonic, allays hysteria and asthmatic complaints, and dissolves polypi." Myrrh apparently prevents the hair from falling out too!.[65]

Mucous Membranes

The *British Pharmaceutical Codex 1934* carries several formulas containing myrrh. In the main monograph it is stated to be 'mildly disinfectant and stimulating to the mucous membranes'. Certainly myrrh has been used to relieve wet asthma due to its ability to reduce excessive mucous membrane discharge. In *The Complete Herbalist* by Dr P. Phelps Brown, Newcastle Publishing, 1872, myrrh is mentioned as a stimulant of the mucous tissues, particularly with excessive secretion and was used to promote expectoration. Myrrh powder and tincture have been subjects of a German therapeutic monograph for the treatment of mild inflammations of the oral and pharyngeal mucous membranes.[66]

Myrrh is an ideal inhalant for bronchial conditions. By deeply inhaling the vapours from a few drops placed on hot water, effective relief can be obtained from spasmodic coughing. Two well-documented cases of the administration of myrrh and frankincense to children with severe bronchial infections were reported in 1991.[67]

The Blood

Steroidal-like compounds extracted from *Commiphora mukal* were tested on blood samples. The result was marked inhibition of platelet aggregation. The authors suggested that this herbal remedy could be used in myocardial infarction and thromboembolism.[68]

Though a number of studies have shown myrrh extracts do have a variety of medicinal actions many of the studies have been concerned with the internal administration of the extracts in animals, so they may not be valid in humans. Different studies have shown: hypolipidaemic and hypocholesteraemic effects, inhibition of platelet aggregation, anti-inflammatory, phagocyte stimulation and thyroid activating activity. *(Delaveau P. et. al. 1980. Planta Medica 40, 49. Malhotra S. et al. 1971. Ind. J. Med. Res. 59 (10). Srivastava M. et. al. 1984. J. Biosci. 6, (3) 277. Mester L. et al. 1979. Planta Medica, 37 (4) 357. Tripathi S. et. al. 1975. Ind. J. Exp. Biol. 13, (1)15.* Myrrh was given internally and was found to lower cholesterol and reduce plaque formation in aortas of rabbits.[69]

Other uses

It seems that myrrh was also helpful in preventing hair loss since we are told that "it prevents the hair from falling". It also makes "a stimulating and antiseptic gargle. It should only be used in small doses".[70]

Myrrh is sometimes looked upon as a uterine stimulant. It has been said to be highly useful in enfeebled conditions of the body and valuable for suppressed menses, and leucorrhoea.[71] However, there is little scientific evidence to prove that myrrh is a uterine stimulant.

An insecticidal activity has been found in some of the natural components in myrrh called *furanosesquiterpenoids*. This research was undertaken after it was found that Somalian herdsmen applied myrrh resins to cattle to deter ticks; simply one more case of modern science proving that these ancient remedies work.[72] In 1995 a study was published on the traditional remedies used in Ethiopia to expel intestinal tapeworms. This study indicated that the resin from *C. resinifula* was an effective preparation for this problem.[73]

The aforementioned studies when taken with traditional usage, suggest that in myrrh resin we have some highly effective natural remedies. Further research is needed to establish which of the many tree varieties yield the most effective extracts and for which conditions. Such academic research then needs to be applied to the cultivation and harvesting of the trees, to ensure greater consistency of medicinal actions. This type of work has been done on other plants and trees which yield commercially important medicinal and fragrance agents, and it could be done for myrrh.

The uses of Myrrh in Aromatherapy

Myrrh is a very sticky resinous substance which is, therefore, used infrequently in aromatherapy massage or baths. However, it is still invaluable as an ingredient for *mouthwashes* especially for problems such as gingivitis and mouth ulcers. It is excellent for sore throats, often mixed with lemon and thyme. Although 90% alcohol is the best medium for dissolving the essential oils this cannot be easily obtained by the public. Some aromatherapists use brandy or vodka as substitutes to partly dissolve the essential oils, to make preparations which might comprise 1 drop thyme, 2 drops myrrh and 2 drops lemon in a teaspoonful of either alcohol, vodka or brandy. This mixture is thoroughly shaken in a 250 ml bottle to which distilled water is added. Unless pure alcohol is used, the essential oils will come out of suspension though the mixture is still quite effective. Instead of distilled water, milk can be used as it is a natural emulsifier.

Myrrh is sometimes used in essential oil *burners* as it adds a very subtle spicy note to an aromatic blend. It is best used whilst it is still fresh since it is then still quite runny. Only a drop need be used as it is very strong and can overpower other essential oils. It blends well with geranium, cinnamon leaf and patchouli.

Ancient Formulas containing Frankincense & Myrrh

These are presented for historical interest and
and **not** recommended for use

Arab Medical Texts of around 750 AD (al-Hindi)

Drug for abscesses for which the lancet is not indicated
Aloe juice, *myrrh*, gum ammoniac, verdigris, equal part of each. Pound together, sprinkle on the wound and cover with a cloth.

For pain from decayed teeth affected by cold
Myrrh is pulverized and sprinkled on the inside and outside of the base of the tooth. This was supposed to bring speedy relief.

A dentifrice to arrest gum shrinkage
Myrrh, cuttle fish bone, borax, equal parts. Pounded and sieved and placed in the gum of the sick one.

Drug for dirty, old, partly healed wound
Plantain pulverized with yogurt and placed in the sun for an hour. Then the wound is smeared with it to make the clot smaller and alive, as it contracts. When gentle heat is introduced, it becomes thinner so that it trickles. It is anointed with *myrrh*, lithage (white lead), which has been pulverized and sieved and rose oil, so that it is cicatrized with speed, God willing. *(This formula does make some sense since it contains plants with astringent, anti-microbial and healing properties, though side effects must have occurred with the poisonous lead.)*

For a wound in the neck
Myrrh one part, with flour of the djbt plant. Work into a mass and bind onto the wound.

For inflamed wounds
Myrrh, burnt resin, cassia and cinnamon.

Drugs for nosebleeds and for a sty
Cobweb is stirred in water with cucumber, *myrrh*, wine vinegar, gum of an old oak? Chinese ink, and amber. It coagulates the blood at the opening of the vessel.

For a cough caused by catarrh
Sugar 2 parts, liquorice 1 part, *frankincense* 1 part, gum arabic 2 parts, gum tragacanth 1 part. All are pounded and sieved and mixed with honey.

SOME 'PEARLS OF WISDOM' FROM MEDICAL TEXTS C. 1450 AD

For headache
1) Blend wormwood, wax and *incense* with the white of an egg. Put it in a linen cloth and bind it about the head.
2) Blend *incense* and pigeon's dung with white flour and an egg. Then put it in a linen cloth and bind it about the head.

For infected wounds
Blend beeswax, verdigris, cobblers wax, *frankincense*, pitch and tar, turpentine, sheep's tallow and fry them in a pan. When it is seethed together, cool and put it in boxes. *(Note: this formula would produce an ointment which was slightly astringent and possibly mildly antiseptic.)*

For gout
Blend pitch, beeswax, *frankincense*, sheep's tallow in even proportions. Seethe them together *(this means heating to boiling)*. Lay it on a linen cloth, lay it to the gout and it shall heal.

To staunch bleeding from a wound
Blend *incense*, aloes, fine wheat flour, an egg then grind until thick. Lay this plaster to the vein that be cut, and do not take it away till thou

knowest the gash be closed together. Another use of this paste was to apply it to the wound over fine hair or spiders' webs.

For migraine

Take a pint of vinegar, half a pint of mustard and an ounce of *frankincense*. Make a plaster thereof and lay it on the neck and thou shalt be whole within three or four times, if it be laid fairly hot. *(Note: a fascinating combination here, the hot elements of the plaster would dilate the capillaries in the skin. If used at the correct time this would probably have normalised the circulation problems which caused the pain of migraine. In addition the emotionally relaxing effects of inhaling the frankincense are very important. Note also the emphasis placed on repeating the application several times in order to obtain relief. Of course, the mustard might have burnt the skin if the application had been left on too long or the skin was particularly sensitive.)*

Formulas from 'The Leechbook of Bold'

The Leechbook of Bold was a collection of medical recipes
of the 15th century and included many recipes for the use of Frankincense.
Some of the recipes are quite awesome.

To quote a rather hair-raising recipe for **blindness** which is, of course,
not recommended: 'A precious water for the eyes, that if a man had lost
his sight ten years, if it were possible he shall recover it gain within forty
days. Take smallage, rue, fennel, agrimony, betony, scabious, avens,
houndstongue, eyebright, pimpernel and sage and distil these together
with a little urine* of a boy-child and five grains of *frankincense*. And
drop that water each night in the sore eyes'.

Another recipe was for **swelling of the body**. 'Take lard, old grease
and sheep's tallow, of each equally as much and take *incense* and wax,
of each equally as much; oil, the third part. And take the root of
hollyhock roasted and well pounded together with the grease and let it
softly seethe and coole it and put it in boxes and put it on a cloth and
lay to the wound'.

A recipe for **leprosy** included the dangerous Mercury. 'Take quick-
silver (Mercury) and boar's grease, and black pepper and *incense*; and
stamp them all together and therewith anoint the face, and keep it from
the wind three days, and it shall be whole'.

For **sore and enlarged nipples** 'mingle the powder of *incense* with
vinegar, and anoint them therewith, and they shall become small'. (Said
to be a very ancient and effective remedy for this condition. This
combination would have strong astringent properties as well as anti-
inflammatory and healing effects).

For **headache**, take *incense* and pigeon's dung, wheat flour, an ounce
of each and temper them with the white of an egg; and whereso the
head acheth, bind it, and it shall vanish anon.

*There are those who would recommend 'urine therapy' today – see
John W. Armstrong's *'The Water of Life'*, pub. The C. W. Daniel Co.

Formulas used by Medical Herbalists

Some may still be in use but they are best left to those
best qualified to deal with them

A fumigating powder to give an aromatic odour to a sick-room
Frankincense 10 grams, benzoin 20 grams, storax gum 10 grams, cascarilla 15 grams, potassium nitrate 5 grams, water 5 grams, alcohol 90%. The potassium nitrate is moistened with the water, the coarse powders are then blended with the alcohol and the mixture allowed to dry. The potassium nitrate allows the powders to smoulder slowly with a glow, rather than burn quickly with flame.

Fumigating powder
Benzoin, *frankincense*, storax, mastic, amber, cascarilla, orris root, sandalwood, all reduced to a coarse powder and thrown upon a heated surface.

Arabian incense powder
All coarse powders of: clove 50 grams, cassia 50 grams, cascarilla 100 grams, benzoin 100 grams, *frankincense* 1000 grams, to be blended and used in an incense burner.

Nepalese incense powder
2 tablesp. *frankincense*, quarter cup juniper leaf, half cup sandalwood, 2 tablesp. cinnamon, 2 tablesp. patchouli, 1 cup and 1 tablesp. powdered cedarwood, threequarters cup water, 1 teasp. potassium nitrate, tragacanth powder as needed.

Nosebleeds
Dioscorides says that 'the juice of leeks mixed with *frankincense* stops blood, especially that which comes from the nose'.

Epilepsy
The lungs of a hare, white wine, *frankincense* and other resins.

Rejuvenating face mask
Live brimstone 1 oz, *frankincense* 2 oz, myrrh 2 oz, ambergris 6 drachms. Powder them severall, then mingle them, adding 1 pint of rose water. Distill them in a double vessel or Bain Marie as they call it. The water distilled from it must be kept in a vessel exactly stopped. When you will use it dip a fine white rag in it and wash your face before you go to sleep, and in the morning wash it off in barley water. The face will be so clear and beautiful that all will wonder and desire to kiss it!

For diphtheria
Fluid extract of Echinacea 1 fl oz, fluid extract of Grindelia camporum 30 drops, fluid extract of calendula officinalis 60 drops, tincture of *myrrh* 20 drops, tincture of hydrastis 30 drops. Add to water to make 8 fluid ounces. Dose: one dessertspoon every three hours.

For quinsy
Fluid extract of echinacea 1 fl oz, fluid extract of calendula officinalis ½ fl oz, tincture of hydrastis 30 drops, tincture of *myrrh* 20 drops. Add to water to make 8 fl ounces. Dose: one dessertspoon every three hours.

An enema
Fluid extract of wild yam 1 fl oz, fluid extract of *myrrh* 20 drops; enema base in water, add to make 20 fl ounces.

For treating diarrhoea and gastro-intestinal bleeding
Coarse powder of catechu 4 fl oz, bayberry bark powder 30 drops, tincture of cinnamon bark 1 fl oz, tincture of Lavender 1 fl oz, tincture of *myrrh* 1 fl oz, alcohol 60% add to make 20 fl oz. Dose: 10–60 drops.

Ointment for old sores
Bayberry wax 1 oz, tincture of *myrrh* 10 drops, gum turpentine 1 oz, olive oil 1 fl oz. Make up as ointment.

A mouthwash formula formerly prepared by Guy's hospital pharmacy
Glycerin of borax 1 oz, tincture of *myrrh* 5 drops, distilled water 1 oz.

A boric acid mouthwash, formerly prepared by the Royal Dental Hospital and St. Bartholomew's hospital pharmacy included:

Boric acid, tincture of krameria, eau de cologne, tincture of *myrrh*.

For obesity
Echinacea and mullein in equal parts, *myrrh* one quarter part. Steep two teaspoons per cup of water for twenty minutes; take quarter cup every four hours.

A liniment for bruises and sprains
Goldenseal, arnica, cayenne pepper and *myrrh* can be soaked in rubbing alcohol for a few weeks to make the liniment.

For consumption
Frankincense dissolved in the yolk of an egg and made into an emulsion with barley-water, will do good in consumptions when almost all other things fail.

Lastly, an extract from *A Kentish Herbal* for wounds, bruises and skin complaints. The recipe to staunch bleeding relies heavily upon old Egyptian corpses.

Take Aloes, *Mirrhe Mummy**, Sandragon of each half an ounce bole Armoniack, Cumfrey Roots, dried Mastick, *Olibanum* each drams iii colophony, halfe an ounce, beat them all to fine powder and searce them, take a little of the poweder and mix it with the whit of an egge beaten & lay it on the downe of A hare and fill the wound with it this powder is fitt to have always in a box by us.

*Interestingly, desiccated Mummy was a much sought after remedy for some time during the Middle Ages and the Renaissance. It was used as a medication against paralysis, weak heart, cough, epilepsy and a host of other ailments. Apparently, it was a Jewish physician named El-Magar, who around 1300 AD, began prescribing a 'mummy' for almost any disease. His practice must have been quite successful because quite soon 'mummy' medication was much in demand. *(The Secret Medicine of the Pharaohs by Cornelius Stetter, Edition Q)*. Genuine mummies were not always easy to come by and no doubt 'substitutes' were often used. Could the real thing have been in any way efficacious? It is not outside the realms of possibility, since the original mummies had been soaked prodigiously in resins and spices, and herbs like rosemary were inserted in the bandages. Yet would the plants' healing properties have remained active over the centuries? Who can tell?

Safety Information

'First do no harm'
Hippocrates c.460

Essential oils of frankincense and myrrh are used extensively in Aromatherapy; frankincense principally in massage and diffusion, myrrh perhaps more in mouth washes and gargles. Its viscous nature tends to discourage application on the skin. These oils are considered quite safe, generally. But we thought it would be of interest to catalogue some published research material on their general application and safety.

FRANKINCENSE

A report to the R.I.F.M. *(Kligman A. 1971)* indicated that an 8% solution of frankincense *gum* and an *extract* from the gum tested on humans showed no sign of skin irritation or sensitisation. However, other experiments have recorded a very small number of undesirable skin reactions following the use of *unrefined* frankincense resin extracts. The use of olibanum (frankincense) in adhesive plasters and in perfumes has also caused dermatitis in sensitive individuals *(Greenberg L. & Lester D. 1954. Handbook of Cosmetic Materials, New York, Interscience). (Schwartz L. et al 1957. Occupational Diseases of the Skin. 3rd ed. Philadelphia. Lea and Febiger, pp.637–672)*.

Frankincense resins have been tested for toxicity and have not been found to represent any dangers to humans, indeed frankincense was approved for use in food by the F.D.A. in America, and *The Council of Europe (1974)* allowed its use in food with a possible limitation of the active principle.

Care should be taken that adverse skin reactions do not occur due to pre-existing allergic conditions.

MYRRH

Myrrh *oil* has been tested for toxicity and has not been found to represent any dangers to humans, indeed myrrh oil was approved for use in food by the *F.D.A.* in America and *The Council of Europe (1974)* allowed its use in food with a possible limitation of the active principles. It is a flavour component of alcoholic and non-alcoholic beverages, frozen dairy desserts, baked goods, gelatines and puddings, meat and meat products *(Encyclopedia of Common Natural Ingredients, A Leung & Steven Foster 1996)*. Myrrh *gum* of the *Commiphora molmol., C. abyssinica* and other *Commiphora* species have actually been listed as safe herbs in a report of the *American Food and Drug Administration (FSA) from 1975 (23)*.

Myrrh *essential oil* tested at 8% solution caused no irritation or sensitisation on human skin. *(Epstein W. 1973. Report to the R.I.F.M.)*. Myrrh *absolute* however, tested at 8% solution caused no *irritation* on human skin, but did cause two *sensitisation* reactions out of 25 volunteers tested. *(Epstein W. 1980 & Kligman A. 1976. Reports to the R.I.F.M.)*. Also adverse dermal reactions have been reported following the use of crude resin extracts. A few reports exist of contact sensitivity to some tree varieties with cross sensitivity confirmed to other balsams.

Conversely, a patient who developed contact dermatitis to benzoin tincture and was then given 18 closed patch tests with various gums, developed a cross-sensitisation reaction to myrrh *gum*. *(Spott D. & Shelley W. 1970. American Medical Association 214 (10) 1881–1882)*. One out thirteen patients contact sensitivity to Balsam of Peru gave a positive patch test reaction to myrrh *gum*. *(Hjorth N. 1961. Eczematous Allergy to Balsams. Munksgaard, Copenhagen)*.

Commiphora gileadense (synonym Balsamodendron gileadense) was suspected of producing allergic effects *(Bardel S. 1935. Les dermatoses par bois toxiques. pp.91)*

The *Commiphora pyracanthoides* species produced a stinging burning sensation on the lips followed by swelling *(Watt J. & Breyer-Brandwijk M. 1962. The Medicinal and Poisonous Plants of Southern Africa. 2nd ed. Edinburgh. E & S. Livingstone)*. It might be advisable therefore, for people suffering allergies to cosmetics and perfumes to avoid the use of myrrh on the skin.

Some very limited animal trials have indicated that extracts from *C. mukul* may have a slight thyroid stimulating effect. Therefore people with overactive thyroid glands should avoid the internal use of myrrh (internal usage of essential oils is not practised by most Aromatherapists).

Provided the appropriate amounts are used, the essential oil can be considered safe, but due to unreliable chemical composition, careful observation should be kept for any sign of skin irritation. Historically, myrrh has a reputation as a uterine stimulant and some people feel this oil should not be used during pregnancy, but there is no sound adverse effects data on this aspect of use. If emmenagoguic properties exist, such action is most likely to be on the internal use of myrrh rather than the external use. *The British Herbal Pharmacopoeia 1983* does not mention this contra-indication.

As with the use of any aromatic substance, it is advisable to suspend their usage from time to time to reduce the slight possibility of the build up of skin sensitisation.

GENERAL

The incidence of adverse skin reactions to most aromatic plants seems to decline with the increasing purity of essential oils extracted from the crude materials. When appropriate amounts are used, trials using resin or essential oils on human volunteers has indicated that the essential oils can be considered totally safe.

Aromatherapists and informed users of essential oils are of course, familiar with the correct applications of oils. For the benefit of people who have never experienced the fragrant delights which these oils can produce, here are a few hints on usage and safety.

Essential oils

– should not be used neat on the skin. For massage blends, one or two drops of essential oil per teaspoon of base oil, like almond, sunflower or grapeseed is sufficient. This advice only applies to frankincense and myrrh as other essential oils require individual assessment of the amounts which may be used i.e. peppermint and thyme may cause irritation at this level of use.

– must not be left unattended with children.

– frankincense and myrrh can be used in heated diffusers, but never leave a candle burner alight during the night and these should not be left unsupervised in a child's room. Myrrh oil is not suitable for cold pumped diffusers as it is too thick and sticky.

– should be kept well away from the eyes.

– must not be left unattended with people who have learning difficulties.

– must not be left unattended with people suffering from loss of manual dexterity.

– should not be kept in bottles that have no fixed dropper inserts. The contents can easily be consumed by a child.

– should not be used on anyone who intends to drive a car or any other vehicle within 15 minutes of being massaged with relaxing or sedative essential oils. This precaution is even more important if the individual is taking medication, social drugs or alcohol, which in themselves may cause drowsiness or reduced concentration.

– containers should be kept upright to discourage seepage of the oil.

– should be kept away from sunlight and heat.

Let common sense prevail when using 'uncommon scents'!

CASE HISTORY: Robert
AROMATHERAPIST: Wanda Sellar

Robert was in his early sixties when he came for aromatherapy treatment. He had a very bad fall some years earlier which put an end to his career. The fall had twisted his pelvic girdle and consequently he was almost constantly in pain. His left knee gave him a great deal of discomfort and he described his calf muscles as 'dead'. He also had severe wind and varicose veins and since the accident experienced difficulty in breathing. Despite all this he was a cheerful fellow and always tried to maintain a positive frame of mind.

After taking his case history, I decided upon essential oils that were analgesic, carminative and helpful to the respiratory and circulatory systems. I therefore chose Lavender to help relax the muscles, Dill as a carminative and Frankincense to help regulate his breathing. After the first treatment consisting of massage using essential oils, he said that his body had felt 'toned up' though he still experienced pain and all the other symptoms. But he felt that aromatherapy had made a difference to his 'well-being' and decided to come for weekly treatments.

By the third treatment he did not feel so bloated and his flatulence had subsided, which pleased him greatly as he had found this quite embarrassing. He also said that he felt more 'balanced' and he described that 'the heat had been restored' to his solar plexus which he felt gave him more energy. Only after his fifth treatment was he able to say that he was no longer in such pain and that his breathing had improved. I had continued using Frankincense in the blend and at times substituted Dill for Ginger to help settle his digestion. As he continued treatment he felt that his muscles felt lighter and he did not feel as if he was 'dragging his body around'. He felt that his digestion and respiration had improved considerably. Naturally since he was breathing better, his body was taking in more oxygen and his organs were working more efficiently.

After weekly attendance for about two months, Robert reduced his attendance to twice monthly treatments and then to once a month for general toning up. Aromatherapy massage and the essential oils had made a difference to his life. He was now in much less pain and could breathe much more easily.

CASE HISTORY: Patrick

Patrick had a very stiff neck and aching back. (He also had other more severe problems for which he was being treated allopathically.) He came for aromatherapy treatment basically for pain relief and to cheer himself up. I therefore chose lavender, bergamot and clary sage to which he responded very well.

Even after the first aromatherapy treatment, the pain had subsided but he attended regularly, since he found massage enjoyable, often coming just for a back and neck treatment. What I found interesting was that Patrick had become quite convinced of the efficacy of essential oils and used them at home in a medicinal and pleasurable capacity. One day he came for his usual back massage and after checking his present state of well-being he informed me that he had just got over a cough and a cold. He had treated himself with an essential oil and I was surprised and delighted to discover that the oil which had worked so well was frankincense!

Frankincense & Myrrh in Perfumery

I cannot see what flowers are at my feet,
Nor what soft incense hangs upon the boughs,
But, in embalmed darkness, guess each sweet
Wherewith the seasonable month endows
The grass, the thicket, and the fruit-tree wild;
White hawthorn, and the pastoral eglantine;
Fast-fading violets covered up in leaves;
And mid-May's eldest child,
The coming musk-rose, full of dewy wine,
The murmurous haunt of flies on summer eves.

John Keats: Ode to a Nightingale

Early beginnings

The world of perfumery began as soon as man breathed the air and gloried in the odour of nature. For indeed, the earliest sense to develop is that of smell. Our dependency upon it is illustrated by the infant's ability to recognise the smell of its mother from the 6th day of birth; *Isobutyraldehyde*, said to be the malty milk smell that allows the infant to find the nipple of its mother, and to the source 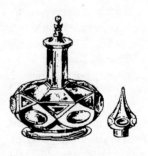 of its survival.[74] The sense of smell informs us as to the nature of things, anticipated happiness or danger. It is quite possible that ancient man's existence depended upon his ability to smell out food, potential mates and lurking predators.

It is believed that the interest in aromatics followed upon the discovery and use of fire. Perhaps our ancestors found that parts of smouldering plants gave off pleasant aromas. Such odoriferous materials might have included sandalwood, cinnamon bark, aromatic roots, vetiver and resinous substances like benzoin, frankincense and myrrh. As the art of perfumery developed, such plant materials would form the central part of fragrances that today we might describe as 'heavy' or 'sombre'.

Before aromatics were valued for personal adornment, they were burned as incense in reverence to the gods. Burning incense was a custom based on what appeared to be a universal belief that the gods had power to control nature and man's destiny. Omnipotent as the gods were deemed to be, their judgement could be influenced by worship and sacrifice, so it was thought. The aromatic smoke accompanying the sacrifice was thought to carry the prayers and supplications heavenward. The practice of burning incense developed rapidly and the art of perfumery seems to have evolved from religious observance. The Latin expression 'per fumum' which means 'through smoke' gives rise to the word 'perfume'.

Arabia led the way into the world of perfumery with the export of gums and resins, though after Petra and Gaza declined as respective centres of the export trade, Constantinople gradually became the main focal point of perfumery. This was around the 6th century AD. Apparently a description of the Saint Sophia cathedral at that time refers to its hundreds of perfume lamps. Perfume ingredients such as frankincense and myrrh were exported to Europe well into the Middle Ages.

It seems, however, that it was the Ancient Egyptians who first systemised documentation of perfume compounds. Some 3,000 years before the birth of Christ, their use for medicinal, cosmetic and ritual purposes was widespread. Some very impressive perfume recipes c.176 BC were found on the wall of the ancient laboratory in the temple of Horus in Edfu, southern Egypt. However, all the Eastern races such as the Chinese, the Assyrians, the Chaldeans, the Babylonians, the Syrians and Persians were experts at making perfumes. Pliny tells us that the first perfumes ought to be attributed to the Persians, for they *'quite soak themselves in it.'* He added that it was just as well since their natural body odour left much to be desired!

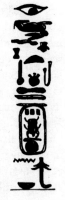

The Egyptians seemed to have been among the earliest to have made the important discovery that if aromatic material is soaked in an oil such as olive, the oil will itself become fragrant. Oils of sesame, balanos, colocynth and even hippopotamus fat were also used as a medium for making perfume.

Woman rolling paste   The perfumes were of course, rather different to those we enjoy today. The essence of plants was extracted by first soaking them in a fixed oil, as mentioned above, then squeezing the mixture through a series of linen bags to produce an aromatic liquid.

Gums and resins were added to ointments and perfumes, not only for their own scent, but also as a fixative for other ingredients. The *kohl* or black powder with which the Egyptian women painted their eyelids, was made of charred frankincense, or other odoriferous resin mixed with frankincense. It was also melted to make a depilatory, and made into a paste with other ingredients to perfume the hands. Cleopatra is said to have welcomed Anthony in clouds of incense.

The range of plants available to the perfumer in ancient Egypt was extensive and included galbanum, cassia, cardamom, cedarwood, angelica, benzoin storax, labdanum as well as frankincense and myrrh. It seems that the Egyptians *may* have known about such animal extractions as ambergris, musk and civet. These give an amazing warmth to perfumes though due to cost and environmental reasons, they are largely synthesised today.

In ancient Egypt, perfumery, healing and worship were aspects of the same magical art. Incense and perfume were lifted to mystical status and the name of *Kyphi* echoes most profoundly throughout the land of the Pharaohs. It was the most celebrated perfume in Egyptian times. Was it the aroma that enchanted the populace? Or perhaps its transcendent quality emanated from its use in worship? Certainly it had some practical uses. Kyphi was an efficient fumigant against rodents, insects and fleas, always plentiful in a hot climate. As a medicine, it was apparently effective in treating lung problems and serpent bites. But maybe its most mysterious quality was its effect upon the emotions. The noted historian, Plutarch (46–126 AD) described Kyphi as being able to *'allay anxiety and brighten dreams'*. Human nature changes little, for we all still have our dreams and the need to be admired and loved is often wrapped up in a whiff of perfume. That was certainly the promise of yesterday and remains the appeal of perfumes today. Ingredients such as frankincense and myrrh are still used in modern perfumes just as they were in ancient compounds such as Kyphi.

Much of the evidence on perfumery in ancient Egypt seems to point to its development by the priestly caste. Yet the book *Disease (Egyptian Bookshelf)*, by Joyce Filer, British Museum Press, p.60 makes an interesting reference to a dwarf named Khnumhotep as being 'Chief of Perfumes' and 'Head of Wardrobe'. Does this indicate that perfumery may not always have been the exclusive province of the priests? Their role as physician would of course indicate that aromatic plants were extensively used in their medicinal ointments and unguents. Making perfumes for aesthetic use would therefore, have been a logical step. Yet it seems that the actual techniques employed in creating perfumes is shrouded in mystery. Also only the crudest kind of equipment is illustrated in Egyptian bas-reliefs, so our imagination has to be our guide as to the intricacies of their labour and expertise.

The Egyptians exchanged their knowledge of perfumery with the Assyrians, Babylonians, Chaldeans, Hebrews, Persians and Greeks, who all developed their own types of perfumes prepared from local plants. Nevertheless, frankincense and myrrh were often included in their perfume compounds.

The earliest mention of aromatic substances in the Bible suggests the importance of aromatic gums. In *Genesis 37:25* when the Ishmaelites came from Gilead with their camels, c.1,730 BC they carried spicery, balm and myrrh. The Hebrews acquired their knowledge in making perfumes from their enforced sojourn in the land of the Pharaohs. The penalties decreed by Moses against the private use of fragrant oils and incense would seem to be proof that the Hebrews, like the Egyptians, used perfumes for their own purposes, chiefly for means of seduction. In *Proverbs 7:17 & 18* we are told:

'I have perfumed my bed with myrrh, aloes and cinnamon. Come, let us take our fill of love until the morning: let us solace ourselves with loves'.

The Old Testament also tells how Esther bathed in myrrh for six months before conquering the heart of Ahasuerus, king of Ancient Persia. *(Esther 2:12)*. Certainly not an advisable practice today!

Ancient Greece and Rome

The Greeks became adept in the art of perfumery and in the preparation of a great variety of cosmetics. In addition to incense, perfumed oils and ointments, believed to have been made by macerating parts of fragrant plants in vegetable oils, they made and used large quantities of fragrant waters. Theophrastus in his treatise 'Concerning Odours, 20–23, says that 'almost all spices and sweet scents except flowers are dry, hot, astringent and mordant (acid). Some also possess a certain bitterness as iris, myrrh, frankincense and perfumes generally.' He goes on to say that the special qualities of myrrh for the creation of perfumes was its ability to 'fix' odours. Whereas most odorous materials/plants faded rapidly, myrrh would last ten years, even improving with age.

Myrrh oil or stacte, was the most durable of any perfume known. Theophrastus informs us that 'from the myrrh when it is bruised flows an oil: it is in fact called 'stacte' (in drops) because it comes in drops slowly...' Once applied to the person, the scent of stacte would linger for some time. Theophrastus also noted that when myrrh was steeped in sweet wine it made the perfume itself more fragrant. Perhaps the most significant perfume at the time of Theophrastus was *Megaleion* which included myrrh among its primary ingredients. Other perfumes of note including myrrh were *Susinon* – the other ingredients were lily, calamus and cardamom; *Amarakinon* also containing cinnamon, spikenard and costus and *Nardinon* which also included spikenard, costus and cardamom. There was also one called the *Egyptian* based on myrrh and cinnamon.

Pliny, the Roman historian c.23–70 AD was also convinced that aromatic gums were indispensable for fixing odour in solid perfumes. 'Indeed,' he is reported to have said 'it (perfume) is apt to die away and disappear with the greatest rapidity if their substances are not employed'. The Romans kept their perfumes or unguents in beautiful containers of alabaster, glass and onyx. *Mendesian* was one of the most famous perfumes containing myrrh at that time. Unguents were either solid, liquid or in powder form. Pliny mentions that 'myrrh even when used by itself without oil makes an unguent, provided that the stacte kind is used'. Pliny also indicated that myrrh was used as an adulterant. A Roman official named Theophanes, travelling in Egypt early in the 4th century AD listed myrrh among his luggage, probably to apply as a lotion after washing.[75]

PERFUMERY TODAY

The fashion in fragrances ebbs and flows with the passage of time. Each age seems to favour an aromatic 'type'. For a time what we might call *'Oriental'* perfumes with their heavy, spicy notes were prevalent in the east. The origin of perfumery in Japan is traced to the practice of Buddhism (introduced there in the 5th century), a religion which requires the burning of incense. The first choice for this purpose was aloes wood but trade with China, Africa, Sumatra and Malaysia, introduced new ingredients for incense burning and perfumery. These were sandalwood, costus root, cinnamon bark, musk, ambergris, fragrant oleo-resins of storax and frankincense.

In the 15th century little caskets contained a variety of spice perfumes like cardamom, saffron, costus, storax and myrrh which were pounded together and made into a paste. The caskets, enclosed in a gold or silver case studded with jewels was pierced with a hole to diffuse the scent. Cardinal Wolsey always carried a pomander in the shape of an orange filled with frankincense.

The discovery of distillation enabled the perfumers to introduce fragrances which heralded lighter, more flowery fragrances. These days perfume compounds fire the public imagination for a decade or so (with some exceptions) only to give way to new and even more exciting creations.

It would seem that aromatics, no longer as necessary perhaps to our survival as in the past, still symbolise a mysterious glamour which seems hard to define. Yet the answer may be quite simple. Aromatics link into the very depths of our emotions since the sense of smell affects the emotional centres of the brain. Odour molecules travel up the nose and quickly reach a sheet of moist mucous bathed tissues – *the olfactory epithelium* – where the molecules plug into receptors located at the ends of stringy structures called cilia. The cilia are outgrowths of neurone molecules, that is millions of sensing cells that collect and transmit information by the nerve fibres to the olfactory bulb which relays the odour message to the limbic system. In humans the limbic system governs sexual behaviour as well as *emotion* and memory which would indicate that our sense of smell is programmed deeply into our memories.

As acknowledged by the ancients, myrrh is an important fixative in perfumes as well as in soaps, creams and lotions. Though myrrh was used extensively in medicine in ancient times, the commercial value of myrrh these days is based upon its use in perfumery. Perfumes are put together with top, middle and base notes. The top notes volatilise quickly so the base notes are next to be added to halt their evaporation. Resins like myrrh were used for thousands of years as what would be called by modern perfumers as a 'base' note. Finally, the middle or heart note is added to a perfume blend in the hope that the result is a balance of perfect harmony.

The odour of myrrh is described as balsamic (warm and sweet) and somewhat spicy-aromatic, sharp and pungent when fresh. Myrrh is employed in modern perfumes as an absolute, oil or resinoid. It is used in Oriental-spicy bases, chypres, woody bases, forest notes and pine fragrances. It blends well, apparently, with geranium, musk, patchouli, spices and the heavier floral bases.[76]

Some modern feminine perfumes including myrrh in their formulations are *Fidji*/Guy Laroche, *Onna*/Gary Farn and *Le*

Jardin/Max Factor;[77] *Le Sport*/Coty, *Opium*/St Laurent (an oriental-type perfume with base notes including myrrh, cedarwood and sandalwood), *Vivre*/Molyneux (a classic floral/aldehyde perfume first presented by Molyneux in the 1930's and relaunched in 1971 with a new formula under IFF); *Eau de Caron*/Caron, *Ispahan*/Rocher, *Alliage*/Lauder (a trend-setting perfume, the green top notes cover a spicy, resinous heart with base notes oak moss and myrrh), *Givenchy III*/Givenchy (an innovative chypre-green perfume with a myrrh base note apparently designed for the career woman) and *Ravissa*/Maurer & Wirtz. In men's fragrances myrrh is found in *Vetiver*/Carven, *Bois de Vetiver*/J Bogart, *Matchbelli*/Matchabelli and *Punjab*/Capucci.[78]

For many people, the smell of frankincense will trigger memories of the incense during attendance at church. Its haunting sweet-spicy smell is described in greater technical detail by Arctander as 'fresh, balsamic, yet dry and resinous, a slightly green odour with a typical, fruit-green top note.' Some say that the oily-green top note is similar to unripe red apples. This is slightly different to the odour of frankincense burnt in ancient temples which may well have been more oppressive. In its resinoid form, frankincense is a valuable fixative, but its distinctive odour is often evident in a perfume blend.

The frankincense resinoid is extensively used in perfumery since the essential oil content of the raw material is only about 8%. Experience in selecting the correct material for distillation or for the extraction of resinoids or absolutes, is a unique and valuable skill. It is partly based upon years of experimenting with the distillation and extraction of all categories of frankincense. Some of the oil is obtained from the dust and siftings of the resinoids but the yield is low and hardly likely to appeal to the discerning nose of the perfumer. Yet there is no exact rule as to which colour of olibanum 'tears' will yield the finest oil, though the quality of the resulting oils is often dependent upon the quality and age of the material. Some indication of the final aromatic quality will be apparent in the odour of the crude botanical material, though only through distillation can the fragrance be truly appreciated.[79]

Oleo-gum-resin ex *Boswellia serrata*, also known as Indian olibanum, yields an essential oil and resinoid which are quite similar in properties to those obtained from commercial olibanum of African origin; though it is considered slightly inferior, examinations have revealed that this is not always the case. These two products have a extensive and varied use in the perfume industry. As discovered by the ancients, modern perfumers agree that the alcohol-soluble resinoid of frankincense has tremendous fixative properties and indeed is among the best fixatives available to the perfume industry. The essential oil and absolute are used as fixatives and/or fragrance components in soaps, detergents, creams, lotions, alcoholic and non-alcoholic beverages, foods generally and perfumes.[80]

The frankincense gum-resin is often used in the preparation of incense powders and sticks. The essential oil has an important place in many styles of perfumes, especially in Oriental perfumes imparting a 'rounding-out effect and alluring tonalities'.[81] It is also used as an Oriental base for some floral perfumes, citrus colognes, spice blends, violet perfumes and in men's fragrances. A exceptional oriental note can be created with sandalwood, vetiver and cinnamon bark oil.[82] It is said to blend well with spice oils, labdanum, mimosa, neroli, muget bases, woody notes and other balsamic notes. Frankincense used in citrus colognes moderates the sweetness of bergamot and orange oils. A similar effect is obtained in the 'fresh' perfume notes such as verbena.[83] (NOTE: ordinary cinnamon bark and verbena essential oils should not be used in formulas for use on the skin. The perfumery trade uses specially treated oils to make their products safe).

The olibanum/frankincense used commercially in the perfume industry and incense manufacture in Europe is imported from Aden, and that used in the United States comes from three countries – India, Eritrea and Somalia. These resins differ in their properties and probably differ also in their botanical origin (species). Perfumers depend on non-specific tests such as colour, odour and acid number or on gas chromatography to test the quality of produce.[84]

The oldest perfume on the market, created in 1889 and now regarded as a perfume classic is *Jicky* by Guerlain, said to include incense as one of the base notes along with vanilla.[85] Some modern feminine perfumes including frankincense in their formulations include: *Replique*/Colonia, *Sculptura*/Jovan, *Mel*/Frances Denney and *Volcan d'Amour*/Diane von Furstenburg.[86] Also *Intreague*/Carven, *Cinnabar*/Lauder, *Soir de Paris*/Bourjois (a fragrance with an incense base note along with vetiver and styrax, which set a trend in the development of sweet floral perfumes.) *Youth Dew*/Lauder, (an innovative oriental perfume, the ingredients emphasising spiciness and balsamic undertones). Some male fragrances including frankincense are *Aqua Brava*/Puig, *Giorgio*/Giorgio, *Jules*/Dior, *L'Homme*/Roger & Gallet and of course *Old Spice*/Shulton, regarded as the progenitor of the modern type of men's fragrances. It was introduced by Shulton in 1937 and has been a top-selling mass-market men's fragrance ever since.[87]

The inclusion of myrrh and frankincense in perfumes continues still and a perfume actually called **Frankincense and Myrrh** is sold by Czech & Speake in Jermyn Street, London.

Mystical
Frankincense & Myrrh

"He saw that there was no mood of the mind that had not
its counterpart in the sensuous life, and set himself
to discover their true relation, wondering
what there was in Frankincense that made one mystical"
'The Picture of Dorian Grey' by Oscar Wilde

Heavenly Incense

There is probably no civilisation in the East or West which has not
valued the inclusion of frankincense in its religious or mystical ceremonies and rituals. The Egyptians, Persians, Babylonians, Assyrians,
Greeks, Romans and Hebrews all attached great importance to its use.
The Egyptian Book of the Dead refers to frankincense as the 'sweat of
the gods fallen to earth', suggesting its mystical powers. Incense, which
almost always included frankincense, was thrown on red-hot charcoals
or burned in a censer whilst the priest uttered a special blessing or prayer.

There were distinct rules for using the censer and special procedures
in creating incense blends. One such celebrated incense of course was
Kyphi, which embodied all the dreams and fantasies of a superstitious
people. Inspired by numerous ingredients including frankincense and
myrrh, it was prepared in great secrecy and the exact formula still
remains a fascinating mystery. The magic formula, so Plutarch tells us,
was to imbue Kyphi with occult powers.

The preparation of this secret blend was accompanied by
incantations from sacred books and the words, spoken aloud, together
with the aroma, apparently had a profound effect on those present. The
task of burning the sacred incense was allotted to a priest or king. Its
potency was such that the ancient Egyptians believed that the souls of
the dead ascended to heaven in the smoke. Indeed, in the 'Book of the
Dead' – the earliest written record of religious and magical ceremonies
– the use of incense is prescribed to safeguard the passage of the
departed in the afterlife.

The instructions for making the incense and holy oil in the Bible, also including frankincense and myrrh, were divinely revealed and shrouded in mystery. Philo Judaeus suggested that the four ingredients of the holy oil – stacte (a form of myrrh), onycha, galbanum and frankincense symbolized the four elements – water, air, earth and fire. The sacred nature of the incense and oil precluded their use by ordinary mortals. Nor were they allowed to emulate the formula. The penalty for doing so was banishment. Frankincense is mentioned at least 22 times in the Bible. It was referred to once as an article of merchandise, three times as a produce of the royal garden of Solomon, but its most frequent reference is in relation to its use in worship.

The Hebrews also placed frankincense on religious sacrifices to augment the sanctity of the offering. To quote from *Leviticus 2:14–16:* …'if thou offer a meat offering of thy first fruits unto the Lord...thou shalt put oil upon it, and lay frankincense thereon...'

The special reverence accorded frankincense and myrrh implied a deeply symbolic gesture in their presentation, along with gold, to the infant Jesus. They were of course, the most precious substances of their day, yet their occult significance apparently revealed the purpose of his life. Gold was said to be for kingship, frankincense was symbolic of holiness and myrrh of suffering.[88] When the body of Jesus was taken down from the cross, it was bound up with spices by St. Joseph of Arimathea and St. Nicodemus. These disciples were said to have used no less than one hundred pounds weight of myrrh and aloes.

A right time for cutting

Frankincense and myrrh were cut during the hot season, when the gum flows most freely. The Romans referred to this period as 'the dog days', an allusion to Sirius, the dog-star – most brilliant of all celestial bodies. 'Sirius' apparently stems from the Greek Seirios signifying a scorching heat, but it is also linked to the Egyptian god Osiris.[89] It was believed that the ascent of Sirius at the same time as the Sun, increased the heat of the day. This was around the beginning of July when the following six to eight weeks were the hottest weeks of the summer.[90] Cutting the trees was avoided during the rainy season.

Pliny *(Naturalis historia XII, 54)* reports that the frankincense tree and those who were entitled to harvest it were looked upon as sacred. At the time of incision they should be pure in mind and body. Contact with women was forbidden. (Indeed, the offering of incense by way of

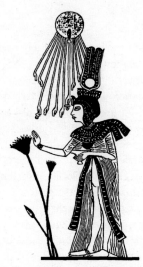

Homage to the Sun — A right time for cutting

purification was offered to couples immediately after sexual intercourse.) It was also prohibited to participate at funerals before taking part in the harvest. Frankincense was considered to be the blood of the tree and so was able to animate the Divine.[91] Together with myrrh it appears in two epigraphic *texts (one CIH 545, Sabaean, the other RES 4336, Qatabanian)* as the name of a god. Though frankincense was associated with holiness and atonement, it was also used for practical purposes in religious ceremonies to 'mask the smell of blood of sacrificed animals'.

The Sacred and the Profane

Incense was apparently favourable to spiritual vibrations due to the smoke rising heavenwards in undulating rhythm.[92] Certainly the alluring sight of incense smoke was a source of inspiration, but its connection to the spiritual world was assisted by the priests' role in a ceremony that was both enticing and mystical. Yet the use of incense was definitely occult in purpose and symbolised the ascent of prayer, spreading of divine influence, showing respect, and effecting purification. Its purifying effect however, may have acted more on the human presence by masking the offending body odours in religious gatherings! This also ensured a protection against evil spirits, fear and negativity, all more likely to manifest in an unpleasant atmosphere.

It would seem therefore, that incense was used either to commune with the Divine or as a talismanic aid to ward off evil spirits. Indeed, wizards and evil spirits are supposed to avoid sites which smell of the burning of frankincense. A more pragmatic though less beguiling explanation for this is due to the fact that an incense burner with charcoal and frankincense is often found in lavatories in some parts of southern Arabia. The incense is of course burned as an air-sweetener but such places are deemed to be a perfect haunt of the 'jinn' or 'evil spirit'! Fumigation with incense is thought to placate the evil spirits.[93] In the same way a hedge planted with frankincense – take note the *Boswellia Roxb.* species is particularly cited – will prevent bad luck or even bring prosperity.[94]

Spells and spooks

To this day it seems, different blends of incense are burned to enhance the performance of magical rites. Usually incense for sacred fumigations is compounded with various combinations of odorous woods, dried plants, gums and resins blended with honey. The blend is modified in accordance with the nature of the ritual and the particular entity invoked. Incense, supposedly, assists the union between man and spirit. This may be linked to herb magic which is thought to connect one's conscious and unconscious mind to a universal energy pattern reflected in the plant kingdom. Frankincense was specifically a herb of protection, since practising magic opened doors to the discarnate spirits of the astral plane. In the same way it had the ability to purify the tools of magic like magical wands, outline a magic circle and seems to have had an affinity with the precious stone Topaz.[95] The Chinese burned frankincense before consulting their oracle book the *I Ching*. Whether they used frankincense from India or from Arabia is not certain, but trade routes did exist with the Arab world.

Herb spells are supposedly best worked at Full Moon particularly when some entity is to be invoked. However, if the aim is to *banish* or exorcise an evil spirit, the time of New Moon is probably more suitable. A simple spell can be worked by calling in the four sacred directions – the four compass points – and then paying tribute to the Four Elements. Herbs are buried in the earth (the Earth element); flung through the air to the Moon (Air element), cast to living waters such as a lake, pond, stream, river or ocean (the Water element) and burned (the Fire Element) so that the smoke can carry the intent heavenward. Finally upon completion it is important to thank the four directions and actively believe that the spell has been activated. The essence of any herbal or plant ritual lies in the reverence and intent which is brought to it.

Other spells using herbs and plants are much more simple. Carrying a plant like an acorn in the pocket supposedly brings fertility; sweeping an area with juniper helps to clear out negative energies and sage and frankincense are used for their purifying effect particularly when setting up an altar. The great Arabian explorer Freya Stark reported that she had seen incense floating on the top of water carriers where it had been used to 'purify' the water. This may have had a practical purpose though no doubt spiritual cleansing was also involved.

Here are some further recipes including frankincense and myrrh which are designed to attract greater fortune and love into our lives. No guarantees are given of success though!

Aphrodisiac

3 ounces of male frankincense, honey, Chinese cubebs, cinnamon, cloves, coriander seed, cardamoms, ginger, white pepper and a touch of lizard! This was boiled in olive oil and taken internally (not recommended of course).

(The following taken from The Complete Book of Incense, Oils & Brews, Scott Cunningham, Llewellyn Publications, St Paul, MN, U.S.A.)

Abramelin Incense

2 parts myrrh, 1 part wood aloe, a few drops of cinnamon oil. This is burned to contact spirits during rituals or as a simple consecration to sanctify the altar or magical tools.

Altar Incense

3 parts frankincense, 2 parts myrrh and 1 part cinnamon. Burned to purify the area around the altar.

Apollo incense

4 parts frankincense, 2 parts myrrh, 2 parts cinnamon, 1 part bay. This is burned during divination and healing rituals.

Born again incense

3 parts frankincense, 1 part mullein, 1 part chrysanthemums. This is burned when grieving over the passing of a loved one.

House purification incense

3 parts frankincense, 2 parts dragon's blood (if you can get some!), 1 part myrrh, 1 part sandalwood, 1 part wood betony, ½ part dill seed, a few drops of rose geranium oil. This is burned to cleanse the home from time to time or before moving into a new home.

Finally a simplified version of *Kyphi* for all magical rituals. 3 parts frankincense, 2 parts benzoin, 2 parts myrrh, 1 part juniper berries, ½ part galangal, ½ cinnamon, ½ cedar, 2 drops Lotus bouquet, 2 drops wine, 2 drops honey, a few raisins.

Mind over matter

There were of course, many practical uses for frankincense and myrrh but the mystical and occult associations are interesting, though belief in their power may have been no more than a psychological springboard towards peace of mind. In ancient Egypt, frankincense was sacred to the Sun god Re who rose each morning in the form of the physical Sun and revitalized man and nature. Theophrastus writing in his *'Enquiry into Plants' IX. 1v. 4–6* mentions how some sailors greedily took and put on board their ship some of the frankincense and myrrh which they found growing in the country of the Sabaeans in southern Arabia. They had apparently collected the myrrh and frankincense from all parts of the temple of the Sun which was most sacred to the Sabaeans in that region. Frankincense was also used to honour the Sun god Bel by the Babylonians and was consecrated to the Greek sun god Apollo.[96]

As well as its links with spirituality, protection and purification of body and soul, frankincense also seems to have the reputation of

banishing unwanted influences, and was important in the rites of
exorcism. There is even mention of the exorcism of a sick cow with
frankincense.[97] It seems that the protective power of frankincense was
attributed to its smell.

The masculine and the feminine

Myrrh's affiliation to the Egyptian goddess Isis, who
presided over the harvest and healing, may account for
its reputation for bringing peace and healing in times
of sorrow and blessings to difficult situations. It was
also said to be useful in moments of contemplation
and meditation. Myrrh's kinship with pearls is
interesting since they too are connected with sorrow.[98]
Whilst frankincense was sacred to the Sun, myrrh
seemed to have more affinity to the Moon. The Moon
was thought to be the Universal Mother, Isis, the
Moulder of Form, by whom all life was shaped into
manifestation and whose light brought all to birth.
Frankincense and myrrh, therefore, may have been the
embodiment of the Egyptian solar deity Osiris and his
wife Isis, the lunar deity. This implied that frankincense was seen as a plant which invoked the male
aspect of the universe[99] whereas myrrh most probably
refers to the feminine counterpart.

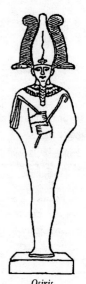

Osiris

A Greek myth may also account for myrrh's association with the
Moon. Myrrha was a beautiful mortal whose mother boasted that she
was lovelier than Aphrodite, goddess of beauty. The vengeful goddess
persuaded the young girl's nurse to entice her into her father's bed – he
somehow remaining ignorant of his new lover's identity. However,
when he discovered who she was, so great was his indignation that he
threatened to kill Myrrha. She fled and he, distraught, took his own life.
As a result of the incest Myrrha became pregnant and in the process was
changed into a myrrh tree. It was the Moon goddess, Diana – also
goddess of childbirth – who pitying the incumbent child split open the
tree. Out tumbled the handsome Adonis who was destined to wreak
such havoc on the affections of young girls. There are other versions of
this myth.[100]

Another fable, according to Herodotus *(II, 73)*, links frankincense
and myrrh to the Phoenix, a fabulous bird who dies and rises from its

ashes reborn. Once in every 500 years the
Phoenix came from Arabia to Heliopolis to bury
his dead father wrapped in myrrh. Pliny records
in his *Naturalis historia (X,4)* that the Phoenix
in his old age constructs for himself a nest of
branches from trees of cassia and frankincense
and fills it with spices in order to die in it. It is
assumed that the legend of the Phoenix was
brought to the Hebrews by south Arabian
traders, and was intended to portray the spices,
which were exported from the frankincense
coast to the whole known world, as a gift of the
gods.[101] Since the myth of the Phoenix refers to
death and resurrection its association with
frankincense and myrrh seems to imbue the trees
and their fragrance with the quality of rebirth.
This very much links into the legend of Osiris

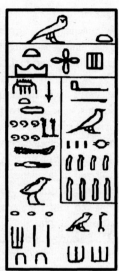

and Isis, since Osiris died and was resurrected through the aid of his
wife Isis.

Incense through the ages

It is interesting that the most common shape of the censer or thurible
was that of a bird, perhaps a symbolic connection to the Phoenix and
rebirth. The symbol of the bird signified *air*, as did incense itself. It was
thought that all four elements should be included in worship. Salt was
included to represent earth, the flames of the candles and charcoal
represented fire and water represented itself.

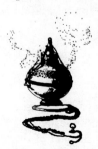

Of course, the *thurible* came in many varieties
and was usually made of very precious materials.
Every religion had its own blend of incense but
frankincense was and is a universally important
ingredient. Frankincense was recommended in the
Anglo-Saxon Leechbooks to be used with myrrh in
the superstitious medical practices of the 11th
century.[102] In the Wardrobe accounts of Edward I,
there is an entry under date 6th January 1299 for
gold, frankincense and myrrh offered by the king
in his chapel on that day, it being the Feast of Epiphany *(Liber
quotidianus Contrarotalutoris Garderobae. Edward I, London 1781.*

pp.xxxii. and 27). The custom is still observed by the sovereigns of England, and the Queens oblation of gold, frankincense and myrrh is still annually presented on the Feast of Epiphany in the Chapel Royal in London *(London 1781, pp.xxxiii and 27).*

In the East incense is used at practically all public worship, whilst in the West, it is often used at High Mass, Benediction, Vespers and Funerals. There is no fixed formula for the incense now used in the Christian churches but frankincense is often the main ingredient in its composition, together with benzoin and storax.[103] In Rome frankincense is the dominant note in incense compounds whereas benzoin is chiefly employed in the Russian Orthodox church. In Lamaism (the Mahayana form of Buddhism of Tibet and Mongolia) frankincense is also employed and the censer resembles that usually used in the Western Catholic church.

Uncertainty about the biological identity of any of the varieties of frankincense in commercial use has led to great confusion regarding their very real difference. This has sometimes made it difficult to obtain the best material for the particular usage required. This dilemma is especially true it seems, with regard to the production of church incense. Church incense manufacturers, ignorant of the differences, sometimes purchase a cheaper or a more readily available variety of frankincense known as 'Indian olibanum'. The odour resembles turpentine or burning rubber when thrown on charcoal much to the displeasure, it seems, of the consumers.[104]

The purifying and protective aspect of frankincense is still evident in some parts of Hadramawt in southern Arabia where the burning of frankincense is performed by someone guilty of a crime. By this action, the tribe is saved from possible disaster. There is a similar custom performed in the Ethiopian church service where the confession of sin over frankincense is part of the rites leading to the celebration of mass.

Astrological Practices

The enchanted formula which produced Khypi was apparently based on a 4 x 4 combination,[105] which totals 16 and reduces to the mystical number 7. This number has an affinity with Neptune, the god of the sea and the planet in astrology signifying spirituality, mysticism and sacrifice. Interestingly, myrrh is said to have been the perfume of Poseidon (the Greek god comparable to Neptune) and the sea nymphs, the Nereids.[106] The planet Neptune however, was not discovered until the 19th century so the association remains an interesting conundrum.

The planet which has associations with myrrh and frankincense, as well as gold, is of course the Sun[107] which also rules the colours yellow and gold – shades of the amber-like 'tears'. In medieval medicinal practices, the Sun was 'hot and dry' as were the plants it was said to govern. Certainly myrrh and frankincense grow in exceedingly hot areas of the globe but their action in healing tends to be anti-inflammatory. It may well be that the oils/resins are imbued with the *Vital Spirits* attributed to the Sun in medical astrology.

The ancients turned to astrology to provide a theoretical basis of disease and to determine why certain plants were efficacious in its

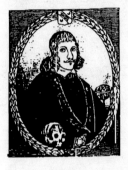

treatment. Indeed, Nicholas Culpeper (1616–1654) tells us that 'physic without astrology is like a lamp without oil'. A very successful herbalist, he used astrology as a guide in choosing the correct medication. His knowledge was taken from the ancient Greek and Arab physicians. Medical astrology is a very complex art but briefly, the position of the planets in the heavens indicates which plant was helpful in healing the disease. If the Sun for instance, signified the medication, this meant that Solar herbs and plants, like frankincense and myrrh, might be used to effect a cure.

Modern mysticism

Current esoteric literature on the magical qualities of gold, myrrh and frankincense seems to echo ancient beliefs. Alice A. Bailey, the founder of the Arcane School of esoteric knowledge, suggests that the nature of man is three-fold: *Physical, Emotional* and *Mental*. Gold, myrrh and frankincense are apparently symbolic of these three levels which have to be 'offered in sacrifice, worship and as a free gift to the *Christ within*'.

Gold, we are told, is a symbol of our physical or material nature, which should be used in service to man and also consecrated to the service of God. Frankincense, on the other hand, represents our emotional nature, with its aspirations, wishes, longings and dreams. These desires are apparently inherent in all nations; the struggle for the expression of these dreams which rise as incense to the feet of God.

Incense is a symbol of that purifying force which removes the debris in our lives and leaves only what is important for the blessing of God.

Myrrh signifies bitterness and relates to the mental nature or the mind. It is apparently through the mind that we suffer as human beings. The further the human race progresses, the more the mind develops and the greater it seems is the capacity for suffering. Yet we are led to believe that suffering is not in vain. When suffering is seen in its true light and dedicated to Divinity, it can be used as an instrument whereby we approach nearer to God. Then we can offer to God that rare and wonderful gift of a mind made wise through pain, and a heart made kind through distress and through difficulty surmounted.[108]

It would seem therefore, that frankincense and myrrh, along with gold, have always been symbols of some inner need to commune with the 'Gods', nature or our higher selves.

GLOSSARY

ABSOLUTE A refined aromatic extract from plant material which is produced by dissolving out the aromatic compounds from the 'concrete' with solvents.

ACCORD A harmonious blend of a number of aromatic materials.

ALDEHYDE An important group of chemicals derived from some natural plant materials.

AL-KINDI, YAQUB A famous Arab philosopher and physician who wrote the celebrated book 'Book of Perfume Chemistry and Distillations'.

ALUM Aluminium potassium sulphate – a powerful astringent used widely in medicinal preparations in the past.

AMBER Another name for ambergris (ambra) a substance excreted by the sperm whale and used in perfumery. Not to be confused with the Amber oil from fossilised pine resin.

ANALGESIC Relieving pain.

ANTIBACTERIAL A substance that stops bacteria growing (Bacteriostatic) or that kills them (Bacteriocidal).

ANTIMICROBIAL Applies to any infectious organism.

ANTISEPTIC Counteracting infection.

ASPERIGILLUS A genus of moulds.

ASTRINGENT Constricting skin tissue.

BALSAMIC A fragrance characterized by a soft warmth and sweetness.

BASE NOTES 1) A term used for the foundation of a perfume composition. 2) An aromatic material/plant whose aromatic molecules diffuse slowly, thus having the power to prolong or fix a fragrance. Frankincense and myrrh were valued for this quality.

BDELLIUM An aromatic gum obtained from some species of the genus Commiphora (or Balsamodendron) which comprises myrrh and opopanox.

CHYPRE NOTE A French word meaning 'Cyprus' and in perfumery it refers to a perfume using Oakmoss, Sandalwood, Musk, Rose, Jasmine and citrus aromatics.

CONCRETE A fatty aromatic material obtained from plants by extraction with solvents.

CUNEIFORM A tablet on which is written wedge-shaped characters of various ancient languages of Mesopotamia and Persia.

DIOSCORIDES A Greek army physician, producing the famous 'Materia Medica' c. 78 AD which included accounts of natural medicines and perfumes.

DISTILLATION The process of transforming a liquid or solid into the vapour state and then condensing the vapour back to its original state.

ELECTUARY A paste taken orally usually containing honey or syrup.

EMMENAGOGUE Stimulating onset of menstruation.

ENEMA A traditional method of administering medicines via the rectum.

ESSENTIAL OIL An aromatic volatile liquid obtained by extraction from an aromatic plant by distillation or other methods.

EUPHORIC Promoting a feeling of well-being and relaxation.

FIXATIVE A substance which will promote the retention of the fragrance on the skin for a lengthy period of time.

FIXED OIL A plant oil comprising mixtures of fatty acids which may be solid at room temperature.

FUMIGATE To treat with smoke something contaminated/infected.

GALLNUT Formed by an insect on the leaves of oak trees, forming an ingredient of ancient perfumes.

HEAVY NOTES Referring to the least volatile ingredients in perfumes, giving a dominant effect.

HERODOTUS A Greek historian b. c 485 BC who wrote 'The Histories' in which he includes perfumes of antiquity and information about the trade in frankincense, myrrh and other resins and spices.

HEXANE Chemical solvent.

HIPPOCRATES Greek physician, c.400 BC known as 'the father of modern medicine'.

HYPOCHOLESTERAEMIC Lowers the level of cholesterol in the blood.

HYPOLIPIDAEMIC Lowers the level of all blood lipids (fats).

IMHOTEP Egyptian physician and architect to Pharaoh Djoser for whom he built the first pyramid in c.2630 BC. Imhotep was later raised to the status of a god.

IN VITRO Biological processes/reactions carried outside the organism in artificial conditions.

IN VIVO Biological testing carried out on or in the living creatures.

LABDANUM An oil or gum from Cistus Ladaniferus – the oil is also called Cistus.

LAVANDIN A hybrid of lavender.

LIMBIC SYSTEM The part of the brain governing feelings, emotions and other basic functions.

MACERATION An age-old method of obtaining aromatic substances from plants by placing them in a non-volatile oil or animal fats.

MIDDLE NOTE Aromatic material of intermediate volatility.

OLEO GUM RESIN A plant extract consisting of a mixture of essential oil, water-soluble gum and resin.

OLEO RESIN A plant extract consisting of a mixture of essential oil and odorless resin.

ORIENTAL FRAGRANCE A perfume which is naturally heavy and long lasting and generally reminiscent of the East.

PHAGOCYTE A cell which has the power of destroying harmful-micro-organisms in the blood.

PLATELET A minute particle in the blood involved in clotting of the blood.

PLINY Born Gaius Plinius Secundus in Northern Italy in AD 23, and known as Pliny the Elder. He is an important source of information regarding the incense trade.

POLYMERISATION A process occurring naturally in certain essential oils where with age the molecules stick together to form a substance similar to plastic.

PURGATIVE A strong laxative.

RE or RA The Sun god, who traveled in the sun barge over the heavens and rose each morning heralding a new day.

RESINOID A term used in perfumery denoting a resin washed with chemical solvents or alcohol to remove sticky soluble materials and the water soluble gum.

R.I.F.M. Research Institute for Fragrance Materials. This is an International organisation of the fragrance trade based in the USA. They test and publish the results on most commonly available fragrance ingredients.

SHERD Or 'Shard' refers to broken bits of pottery.

SPASMOGENIC Relaxing nervous tissue.

STACTE Myrrh in Greek, meaning 'it comes in drops slowly' according to Theophrastus.

STAPHYLOCOCCUS AUREUS Pus-producing bacteria.

STEAM DISTILLATION A process of extracting essential oils by passing steam through plant material.

SYNERGISTIC The combined action of groups of compounds producing a superior effect to each single substance.

THEOPHRASTUS born 370 BC in Lesbos, physician and botanist, who was interested in the classification of plants. He wrote 'Enquiry into Plants'.

TINCTURE An alcoholic extract from natural products.

TOP NOTES An aromatic material giving the first fragrance impression usually of high volatility.

UNGUENTS Ancient name for a semi-solid ointment, obtained by steeping plant material into animal fats.

VISCOUS A gummy, thick and sticky substance.

VOLATILE A substance which evaporates when exposed to the air.

LEBONAH

a 'meditation oil' especially blended by the authors
to invoke the past and capture the present.

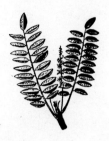

This exclusive blend of essential oils including frankincense,
was designed specifically for use in incense burners,
or in heated essential oil diffusers.

The blend of oils chosen provides a wonderful aroma, neither too
relaxing or too stimulating.

A fragrance for contemplation.
A fragrance for meditation.
A fragrance for the spirit.

FOR DETAILS SEND A **STAMPED** A5
SELF ADDRESSED ENVELOPE TO:

**Lebonah
7, Elm Court Park
Chelmsford Road
CM4 OSE
UK.**

**If you live in the U.S.A. write to:
Sylla Shepard-Hanger
The Atlantic Institute of Aromatherapy
16018 Saddlestring Drive
Tampa
FLORIDA 33618**

THERAPEUTIC INDEX

The following index is not intended as a guide to potential self medication. There are certainly some conditions in the index that are amenable to self treatment. However any unusual or persistent conditions should always be diagnosed by a doctor, before embarking on self medication.

A modern Medical Herbalist would rarely use frankincense or myrrh alone. Rather each patient would receive an individualised medicine, with a number of ingredients aimed at correcting the whole metabolism. If you feel the information provided in this book may help an ailment that you are suffering from, then please do bring the information to the attention of any Herbalist that you consult.

APPENDIX

Notes

[1]*A Modern Herbal, Mrs M Grieve, Tiger, 1992 (various editions available)*

[2]*Nigel Groom (Frankincense & Myrrh, Longman 1981) quotes Gleuck 1939*

[3]*Frankincense & Myrrh, Nigel Groom, Longman 1981*

[4]*Cf.G. Caton Thompson, The Tombs and Moon Temple of Hadramawt Oxford 1944, p.50f. and 16f.*

[5]*Cf. Maria Hofner, 'Die Vorislamischen Religionene Arabiens', in H. Gose, Maria Hofner, K. Rudolph, 'Die Religionene Altsyriens', Altarabiens und der Mandaer (Die Religionene der Menschheit, 10,2), Stuttgart 1970, p263.*

[6]*The Magic of Herbs by C. Leyel 1932*

[7]*Pharmacographia by Fluckiger and Hanbury 1879*

[8,9,10]*National Geographic 'Arabia's Frankincense Trail', Thomas J. Abercrombie, Oct 1985*

[11]*The Secret Medicine of the Pharaohs, C. Stetter, Edition Q 1993*

[12]*Pharmacographia by Fluckiger and Hanbury 1879*

[13]*Tschirch und Stock, Die Harze, Berlin 1935*

[14]*A History of the use of Incense in Divine Worship by E G Cuthbert F. Atchley: Longman, Green & Co*

[15]*A Test of Time, David M. Rohl, BCA 1995*

[16]*Economic Botany 1959. B. Bill Baumann, p.84*

[17]*Perfumery and Cosmetics, George Howard, Arnould-Taylor Education Ltd 1987*

[18]*A Modern Herbal, Mrs M. Grieve, Tiger 1992*

[19]*Notes on the use of Frankincense in South Arabia – Waltr. W. Miller*

[20]*Traditional Astrology magazine, Issue No. 3, 1993*

[21]*G. Ryckmans, de L'or de L'encens et de la myrrhe in 'Revue biblique 58 (1951, p.372–376)*

[22]*Chishull, 'Antiquities Asiaticae', 1728, p.65–72*

[23]*The travels of Marco Polo, Thomas Wright (Ed) Bohn, London, 1899, ch 41 & 42, pp.440–42*

[24]*M. Hartman 'Die Arabishe Frage Mit einem Versuche der Archae-ologie Jemens' (Der Islamische Orient. Berichte und Forschugen, 2,*

Leipzig 1909, p.415f

[25]E. Brauer, 'Ethnologie der jemenitschen Juden', Heidelberg, 1934, p.222f.

[26]H.Vocke 'Die Beschwerde der Addil-Moschee: Eine Satire des jementischen Dictr. Ali Hasan al-Hafangi' in Zeitschrift der Deutschen Morganlandischen Gesellschaft 123 (1973) p.62

[27]Plants of Dhofar 1988. Publ. Adviser for Conservation of the Environment. Sultanate of Oman

[28]Frankincense and Myrrh, Nigel Groom, Longman 1981.

[29]E. Hairfield et al. 1984. Perf. & Flavorist Vol. 9, pp. 33–36.

[30]G. Chiavari et all 1991. J. Ess. Oil Res. 3. pp. 185–185

[31]J. Verghese & M. T. Toy, Flav. & Fragr. J. 1987, Vol.2.

[32]Wilson R & Mookherjee B. 1983. 9th Int. Congr. Ess. oils. Singapore.

[33]Herbal Review, Winter 1982. Frankincense and Myrrh.

[34]The Secret Medicine of the Pharaohs, C. Stetter, Edition Q 1993

[35]The Healing Hand, Majno G. 1975, Harvard University Press

[36]Plants of Dhofar, 1988, Adviser for Conservation of the Environment, Sultanate of Oman

[37]The Useful Plants of Tropical West Africa. M. Dalziel MD.1948

[38]Reddy G. & Dhar S. 1987. Ital. J. Biochem. 36, 4.

[39]Plants of Dhofar, 1988, Adviser to the Sultanate of Oman.

[40]Samuel ben Yozef Yesuca, Nahalat Yosef, Jerusalem 1907.1.p.147

[41]Plants of Dhofar, 1988, Adviser for Conservation of the Environment, Sultanate of Oman

[42]Useful Plants of India. 1873.

[43]C.de Landberg, Datina (Etudes sur les chalectes de l'Arabie meridionale, 2) Leide 1905–1913. p.1308

[44]T. M. Johstone. Folklore and Folk Literature in Oman and Socotra, in Arabian Studies 1, (1974).p.19

[45]Samuel ben Yozef Yesuca, Nahalat Yosef, Jerusalem 1907,11. p. 23.

[46]The Useful Plants of Tropical West Africa. M. Dalziel MD. 1948.

[47]E. Rossie., L'arabo parlato a Sana 1939, p.169

[48]W. Phillips, Unknown Oman, New York 1966. p.176.

[49]Meek, Tribal Studies 1. 197. 257.

[50]Atal et al. 1980.

[51]Abdel Wahab S. et al. 1987. Planta Medica. 3. 382–384.

[52]Ammon H. et al. 1993. J. Ethnopharmacology. 38. 113–119.

[53]Kirtkikar and Basu. 1933.

[54]Plants of Dhofar, 1988, Adviser for Conservation to the Sultanate of Oman

[55]Mitchie C. et al. 1991. J. Royal Soc. of Med. V.84. Oct.

[56]*Majno G. 1975. The Healing Hand, pub: Harvard University Press*
[57]*Encyclopaedia of common natural ingredients by A Leung & Steven Foster 1996.*
[58]*Disease (Egyptian Bookshelf), Joyce Filer, British Museum Press, 1995*
[59]*Frankincense & Myrrh, Nigel Groom, Longman, 1981*
[60]*Solvason H. et al 1988. J. Immunology, 140, 661–665*
[61]*Claeson P. and Samuelson G. 1989, Phytotherapy, Res 3.5–180–185.*
[62]*Unpublished trial: Majno G. 1975. The Healing Hand, pub: Harvard University Press*
[63]*Arora R. Et.al. 1972. Ind. J. Med. Rs 60. 6th June. 929–031 and 1971. 9 (3). 403–4.*
[64]*McDowell P. Et al. 1988 Phytochemistry. 27.8.2519–2521*
[65]*Leyel C. 1947 Compassionate Herbs, pb. Faber & Faber and Leyel C. Herbal Delights.*
[66]*Monograph Myrrh, Bundesanzeiger, no. 193 (Oct 15, 1987).*
[67]*Michie C. & Cooper E. 1991. J. Royal Soc. Med. Vol 84, October 602–605.*
[68]*Mester L. et al. 1970. Planta Medica. Vol.37.367–369.*
[69]*Bensky D-date unknown-Chinese Herbal Medicine*
[70]*Leyel C. 1947 Compassionate Herbs, as above*
[71]*The Complete Herbalist by Dr P. Phelps Brown, Newcastle Publishing 1872*
[72]*Asafu Maradufu 1982. Phytochemistry Vol. 21. No. 3, 677–680).*
[73]*Belachew D. 1995 J. Ethnopharm 45. 27–33.*
[74]*Scents and Sensuality, Max Lake, John Munday, 1989.*
[75]*Frankincense and Myrrh, N. Groom, Longmans, 1981*
[76]*Perfume and Flavor Materials of Natural Origin, S. Arctander, By kind permission of Mr. S. Allured of Allured publishing Corp. 362, South Schmale Road, Carol Stream, Illinois, USA.*
[77]*Fragrance Foundation 1983.*
[78]*The H and R Fragrance Guide, Gloess Publishers and The Perfume Handbook N. Groom, Chapman & Hall, 1996*
[79]*S. Arctander as 76.*
[80]*A. Leung and S. Foster (1996), Encyclopaedia of Common Natural Ingredients in Food, Drugs and Cosmetics. J. Wiley and sons.*
[81]*Arctander as 76 above.*
[82]*Arctander as 76 above.*
[83]*Arctander as 76 above.*
[84]*A Rapid Test for the Identification of Incense Resins. E. Hairfield et al. 1984. Perf. & Flavorist Vol. 9. pp. 33–36*
[85]*The Perfume Handbook, Nigel Groom, Chapman and Hall, 1996*

[86]*Fragrance Foundation 1983.*
[87]*The Perfume Handbook, Nigel Groom, Chapman and Hall, 1996*
[88]*The Occult Properties of Herbs*
[89]*The Fixed Stars & Constellations in Astrology, Vivian E Robson, Aquarian Press 1923*
[90]*The Herbal, John Gerard 1633 edition and Theophrastus, Enquiry into Plants, IX. 1.4–7*
[91]*W. R. Smith in Lectures on the Religion of the Semites, Tübingen, Germany 1899, p.327*
[92]*The Science of the Sacraments, C. W. Leadbetter, Madras 1929*
[93]*D. B. Doe and R. H. Sergeant, A fortified tower house in Wadi-Jirdan in Bulletin of the School of Oriental and African Studies 38 (1975 pl. 5)*
[94]*The Useful Plants of Tropical West Africa, M. Dalziel MD. 1948*
[95]*The Master Book of Herbalism, Paul Beyerl, Phoenix 1984*
[96]*The Master Book of Herbalism, Paul Beyerl, Phoenix 1984*
[97]*The Geographical Handbook, June 1946, p.431*
[98]*The Master Book of Herbalism, Paul Beyerl, Phoenix 1948*
[99]*The Master Book of Herbalism, Paul Beyerl, Phoenix 1948*
[100]*Zimmerman 1964*
[101]*F. Homel, Der Gestirndienst der alten Arber und die altisraelitsche Überlieferung, Munich 1901, p. 12*
[102]*Cockayne, Leechdoms of Early England ii (1865) 295, 297*
[103]*A Modern Herbal, Mrs. M. Grieve, Tiger 1992*
[104]*A Rapid Test for the Identification of Incense Resins, Elizabeth Hairfield etc. Perfume and Flavours, Vol. August/Sept.1984., Allured Pub. Corp.*
[105]*Compassionate Herbs, Mrs. Leyel*
[106]*The Book Perfume, Elizabeth Barille and Catherine Laroze, Flammarion 1995*
[107]*Christian Astrology, William Lilly, Regulus, 1647*
[108]*From Bethlehem to Calvary, Alice A. Bailey, Lucis Press 1937*

INDEX